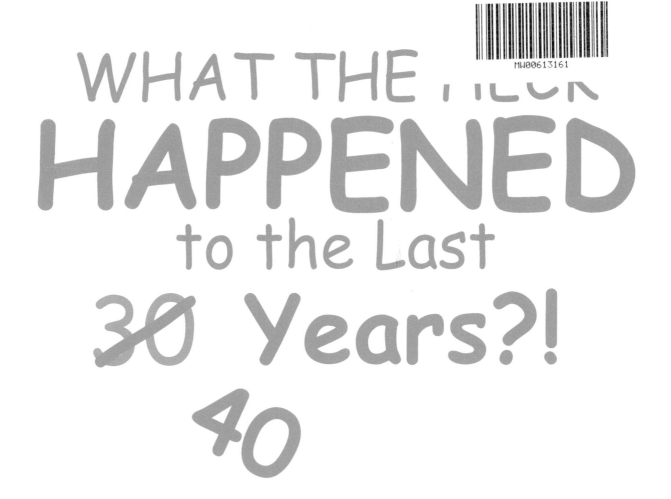

WHAT THE HECK HAPPENED to the Last 3̶0̶ Years?! 40

Robin Dohrman Ayers

Illustrations by Glenna-Jean Alt

NEWMAN SPRINGS PUBLISHING
320 Broad Street
Red Bank, NJ 07701

First originally published by Newman Springs Publishing 2022

Disclaimer: I am not a medical professional, nor do I pretend to be. But I collect a lot of useful information from those who are. Plus, as I have worked with kids with multiple disabilities (and for those who find that not politically correct, when I worked, it was) for thirty years and a sprinkle of adults with like skills, some of the experiences exposed me to similar issues in a variety of ages. However, the crowning start to this idea came from having my mother live with us in her last 7 years and my sister-in-law arriving with end-stage cancer shortly after my mother died. It was a mighty busy bedroom. My viewpoint of one in her 80s and another in her 70s, while I was in my 60s, gave me quite a range of unpreparedness and unanswered questions. And the wee voices in my head pushed me along.

ISBN 978-1-63881-672-0 (Paperback)
ISBN 978-1-63881-673-7 (Digital)

In honor of your fortieth birthday, to Ian, for being a constant source of inspiration all those years.

Contents

Preface

Today at the drugstore, the clerk was a gent.
From my purchase, this chap took off 10 percent.
I asked for the cause of a lesser amount,
And he answered, "Because of the senior's discount."
I went to McDonald's for a burger and fries,
And there, once again, got quite a surprise.
The clerk poured some coffee which he handed to me.
He said, "For you, seniors, the coffee is free."
Understand I'm not old; I'm merely mature.
But some things are changing, temporarily I'm sure.
The newspaper print gets smaller each day.
And people speak softer... Can't hear what they say.
My teeth are my own (I have the receipt),
And my glasses identify people I meet.
Oh, I've slowed down a bit...not a lot, I am sure.
You see, I'm not old...I'm only mature.
The gold in my hair has been bleached by the sun.
You should see all the damage that chlorine has done.
Washing my hair has turned it all white.
But don't call it gray...Saying "blonde" is just right.
My friends all get older...much faster than me.
They seem much more wrinkled from what I can see.
I've got character lines, not wrinkles, I'm sure.
But don't call me old... Just call me mature.
The steps in the houses they're building today,
Are so high that they take your breath all away.

And the streets are much steeper than ten years ago.
That should explain why my walking is slow.
But I'm keeping up on what's hip and what's new,
And I think I can still dance a mean boogaloo.
I'm still in the running… In this I'm secure.
I'm not really old… I'm only mature!

(This is from my late mother's clippings and snippets. Even with MS, she made it to age 87 by sheer determination, Irish spirit, and stuff like this!)

What makes you feel old is when you find out that your friends—people you've known for a long time—are getting brain tumors, suffering through cancer and treatments, and DYING, for Pete's sake! I feel too young to be this old! WHAT THE HECK HAPPENED TO THE LAST 40 YEARS! I didn't see it coming! Old was for my parents.

It's we, the BABY BOOMERS! We're the next line of defense! Most of the proud GREATEST GENERATION is gone, and many of the Silent Generation are now, well, silent. GENERATION X is hot on our heels. But we, the BOOMERS, are marching steadily toward that last line / light / God. Now what? How do we prepare? What should we expect? What words of wisdom should we leave for the ones following—the Gen Xers, the MILLENNIALS, Gen Zers, and the Gen Alphas?

The United States is an aging population. (Ali Velshi, journalist, MSNBC, January 13, 2020)

Those were the days my friend
We thought they'd never end
We'd sing and dance forever and a day
We'd live the life we'd choose
We'd fight and never lose
For we were young and sure to have our way
La la la la la la
La la la la la la
La la la la la

La la la la la la
(Mary Hopkin, Welsh singer/songwriter, 1968)

When you're a child, you want to be a teenager. When you're a teenager, you want to be an adult. When you're an adult, you want to be a cat. (Facebook)

It's very confusing when mentally you feel one age, but your body has gone way ahead of that. We need to find some middle ground! (Vanessa, age 35)

While the average US life expectancy for 2019 was 78.87 years, according to **Macrotrends**, this unfortunately reflects several years in a downhill trend. Despite the US spending the most on health care per capita than any other country in the world, drug overdoses, suicides, alcohol-related illnesses, and obesity are largely to blame.

US life expectancy is still on the decline. (Jen Christensen, CNN, November 26, 2019)

However, from *Parade*'s Paula Spencer Scott, January 12, 2020, comes this informative article, "LIVE HERE AND LIVE TO **100**!" suggesting that one can live in certain cities called Blue Zones, so named by Dan Buettner, a *National Geographic* fellow who has studied societies with the "longest-living people." These groups have high-quality health care; good-for-you, plant-based food; supportive social communities; and healthy, active lifestyles. They are areas "that see older people as assets." Despite problems in the US, the article gave 7 spots which fit most of these characteristics:

1. Southern California beach cities—stress walking and healthy eating with support from local eateries and grocers
2. Breckenridge, Colorado—emphasizes "outdoor motion" and has the "US's longest life expectancy" of 86.8 years as compared to the national average of 79 years (writer's note—unless you break your neck skiing).

3. Minneapolis, Minnesota—provides great health care and thirty farmers markets, nearly the most per person in the nation.
4. Naples, Florida—has high quality health care, lots of leisure activities, multiple housing, and community supports and, for 4 years, has held the title of "healthiest eaters" in a Gallup index.
5. Portland, Maine—stresses continued learning throughout one's life and provides low-cost classes to those over 50.
6. Charleston, South Carolina—number 1 for plant-based eating and lots of land and water activities year-round; and 7 in 10 households have dogs, which equal to more outside time and companions who (yes, I know many people feel this should be *which*, but my pets are *whos* with personalities) lower stress and reduce loneliness
7. Pittsburgh, Pennsylvania—Besides being high on the scale for health care, community, and culture, it has the Age-Friendly Greater Pittsburgh Action Plan focused on moving forward many more beneficial innovations for aging folks. It is also the third most "livable city," following Honolulu and Atlanta, according to one global research group.

Surely the byproducts of COVID-19 in the years 2020/21 will affect the above-mentioned cities. Several were even "hot spots" for the virus. However, with the healthy practices for which they were noted, perhaps they will emerge relatively unscathed. The truth remains to be seen.

I've always been enamored by these inspirational words said by someone—or many ones, probably—in some context, meaningful I'm sure: the secret to getting old is simple—just don't die! Before retirement, I thought that was a good idea. Since entering the ranks of the aging leisure class, though, my attitude has changed a bit. That just-don't-die mode turns out to be pretty boring. Passivity, as attractive as it seems prior to arrival, isn't all that rewarding as a day-in/day-out strategy. In my experience, the great difference between the working me and the retired me has been a sense of purpose. The working me had no problems identifying and describing my purpose. The retired me struggled with that for a while. I discovered that, if one is unable to find or latch onto "purpose" in retirement, quality of life can suffer. At some point—soon, I think—I'm going to quit basing my self-definition on work status—retired versus working. Instead, I've begun to understand myself as being in the third phase of life. Maybe we can agree that the first phase is "Surviving Stupid" or some other title that more befittingly describes the accrual of life experiences sufficient to propel us from adolescence to some modicum of maturity. The second phase might be along the lines of "Saving the World," where we get to do fun things like procreate, cultivate, recreate, and a bunch of other -ate words in order to grow, improve, preserve, and pass along this place to the next generation. I'd like to think the next, and my current, phase might be the "Be That Wise Elder" phase where purpose becomes simplified and is best described as living in the moment, doing today what we might not be able to do tomorrow, and worrying less about what's to become of me while enjoying opportunities to assist others to become the most they can be. I recognize that it would have been nice had I recognized the value of being present in and to the moment in those earlier phases, but I'm also able to appreciate that the moments are now more my own than they might have been in earlier times in life. (Terry, age 68)

Vignette

Terry, as you can see, is well able to compose his own charming version of everything, which I will just quote. Additionally, though, we have been cherished friends from grade school through junior college, then supporters through marriages and losses and a grandchild each, with a span of 40-ish years between; and now we're facing retirement and aging out at the same time. Both sets of parents are gone, and we are making the steady march through our 60s toward that end light together from afar. However, a great difference exists between us. Terry has faced each stage, including great pain during 9/11, with an effervescence that only subsides for a short time to return to its exuberant self. He files but never forgets. I forget but never file and seem to never totally resolve.

Without more adieu, here's Terry:

Well, let's see. People have referred to me in a lot of ways—some earned, some honorific, some affectionate, and some just plain nasty (those I tend to ignore). The most common titles include reverend, doctor, chaplain, colonel, professor [writer's note—show off]. My most favorite titles are son, brother, hubby, dad, pappy, uncle, and friend. Recently I've graduated to the realm of old fart.

And that's Terry.

However, if you find that you must "bloom where you are planted," for the moment, using what you've got left, perhaps you may find some helpful hints, anecdotes, and wisdom for negotiating your aging process—until you are able to or inclined to make a move to one of these live-to-100 cities.

Acknowledgments

It is with the utmost respect and appreciation that I would like to thank the following people for their assistance on this project:

Charlie See (my big brother-type person) for constantly supporting, encouraging, proofreading, and telling me this is in "true Robin style." And thank you for finding Newman Springs for me!

— Darrah (Do) Speis for giving me that one last loving, affirming push into this and making me believe I could do it.
— Kenny Ayers (my husband) whose always, every time, unchanging care about this project many times propelled me through a block or wall that had slowed me down/stopped me. If I said I was going to work on "the book," he took care of everything else and never questioned the use of my time. I'm anxious to see his face when he actually has it in his hands.
— Diana Fritts (my dear friend) who tolerated my running things by her...a lot and incessantly talking about "the book" for oh, three or four years. She also is the person who said (perhaps I'm paraphrasing), "It'll keep her busy and off the streets."
— Our Kathy Puhalla (part of our adopted family) for being the bearer of constant positivity, unconditional love, and encouragement.
— Dr. Neil Crowe for providing the scientific explanation of how thirty years could morph into forty in such a short time.
— Glenna-Jean Alt, whose artwork brought this book to life, thank you for revving up the excitement when we hadn't even met till after the writing was finished! By the way, a trumpet will never work as a trombone.
— Diane Pascoe (author of *Life Isn't Perfect, but My Lipstick Is* and *Never Argue with a Weiner Dog*), who showed me evidence proving that even neighbors can be

published authors. And to my college roommate, Linda Wengerd, who connected me with her neighbor, Diane!

— Gretchen Durst-Hall (whom I've known and called Lizzy since she and Ian were in kindergarten) for her bravery even in the midst of her debilitating disease for putting its description, word to paper, for my sharing.

— Lana Bean of Hampshire Review fame for patiently sizing our pictures to suit the need.

— My catkids, who kept me company, sometimes a little too closely on the keyboard, in the window, and on my notes. But those little/big cat feet were purrfect for preventing boredom. I love you, Maggie, Chai, and Curry...move, I can't see the screen.

— All those who patiently answered my questions for "this book" (ha, right, you humored me and probably thought I'd never get there) and gave me a wee quote, or bigger.

— Any others who heaped on the enthusiasm and made me push forward. Do you know what a thrill it's been to have someone ask, "When's THE BOOK coming out??"

— And to Erma Bombeck for being an inspiration. I miss you, but we WILL always have you 'cause you're in print!

Introduction

(OK, do read this, or you won't know what's going on till halfway through the book!)

In 1971, Erma Bombeck, whom I idolized as one of the most brilliant women on the planet, wrote a book titled *if life is a bowl of cherries, what am i doing in the pits*? And the seed, pardon the pun, was planted. She wrote brilliant and hysterical observations on life. I find, 50 years later, that observations still yield some pretty odd, humorous, and crazy stuff (along with the serious from which I cannot unhinge myself) worth writing about. So here I go. Yes, I know *about* is an adverb...

When I was a kid, my parents told me what to do. I worked 30 years, and the boss told me what to do. Now I'm suddenly old (sort of) and don't know what to do! Where are the instructions?

So why did I write this book? I was tired of wandering around in this older world and not knowing how to deal with it. I'd end up with something that I'd never experienced before (usually bodily), yelling, "Where's the danged instruction book for this?"

I've felt much like my lovely 38-year-old hairdresser, Ashlee, who somewhat unexpectedly one day said, "These twins popped out, but I'm still waiting for the instruction book to pop out." (Eyebrow raiser.)

However, wouldn't it have been so nice to have an elder guide that way? Okay, maybe not exactly. That puts us back to the question, Why was this book written?

This is the answer. Many of us need some kind of assistance in maneuvering through our older years or in helping others. The playing field is different. Our bodies have changed, as have our capabilities. Possibly the thinking cap isn't working quite like it used to. I'm finding difficulty with math, and I'm not THAT old! And we may be a bit emotional about the whole affair as we see things differently than we ever have in the rearview mirror and the windshield. Ian, my son, an almost 40-year-old, did not help this when he spent 2 months weekly hammering into my head that I'm in "that" age group and in "poor health" during the early months of the 2020 COVID-19 pandemic. I got the picture all too clearly.

So to quell the sheer panic and rantings and ravings of a madwoman—me—and to keep me occupied and off the streets, as a good friend insinuated, I started observing actions that are different as we age, jokes and truths on Facebook, and wisdom from a variety of age groups and sources. And I wrote a book using facts and figures (real ones); silliness based on the way I observe life, scary a bit; and medical issues that I knew and referenced relative to the physical changes of aging. Now I'm satisfied that there is a guidebook to becoming older. Of course, it doesn't cover all the parts and pieces, but it hits on quite a few issues. It's written in a friendly, homey style so as to not be intimidating.

Because I had retired after 30 years of immersing myself in "my kids" at school and ended my service to older relatives, hopefully I now had time that I've been wasting on gaming (it keeps my brain active, another part of the whole picture, you know); and I wasn't likely to take up knitting or crocheting and so forth.

I pondered and decided that I wanted to write a book—on something—as my age was penetrating my brain, and I wondered in disbelief, "What the heck happened to the last 30—no, wait—**40** years?" I collected answers and "warnings" of what is to come.

Observations and O Noooos!

Not everyone is given the chance to grow old. So, appreciate and thank God for every single day of your life. (Facebook) Amen.

Sometimes you have to let go of the picture of what you thought life would be like and learn to find joy in the story you're living. (Facebook)

Life is a moderately good play with a badly written third act. (Truman Capote, American novelist)

However, AARP is now advertising that "we may spend more than half of our lives over 50!" (Spring 2021)

Believe people when they tell you life goes fast. (Brian, parent, age 51)

Old age comes at bad time. (San Banducci)

So far, this is the oldest I've ever been and the youngest I will ever be. (Facebook)

To give my thoughts on aging at this point is, honestly, that it's a little strange, LOL. It feels like I'm at this stage where I acknowledge that

I'm older each year as around this part of my life I'm introduced to more responsibilities and really beginning a transition into adulthood, but age is not really something I try to define myself with. Though when I do, I see it more as a challenge to do things that people my age don't usually do rather than a construct to be followed, if that makes sense. (My Reggae/Reagan, a wise age 19)

Being called "ma'am" is a little alarming. I resent being referred to as an OLDER woman. And I DETEST being called ELDERLY. But somehow there are undeniable facts when I stop to think of it. My biggest shock was when the target group for COVID-19 emerged…and it was older people starting at age sixty! SIXTY! That group and up was most at risk!

The greatest lesson I have learned in life is that I still have a lot to learn. (Facebook)

When you're happy and you know it, THANK YOUR MEDS.

Careful grooming may take 20 years off a woman's age, but you can't fool a long flight of stairs. (Marlene Dietrich, actress)

You know, we older folks suffer from **TMB—too many birthdays!** (An acronym stolen from my Dr. Heather's mom.)

When your birthday is coming up, you have only 2 choices: (1) get older **or** (2) die. Pick a druther (that's country for "I'd rather").

Five hundred twenty-five thousand six hundred minutes
Five hundred twenty-five thousand journeys to plan
Five hundred twenty-five thousand six hundred minutes
How do you measure the life of a woman or man?
Remember the love
Seasons of love
("Seasons of Love" by Jonathan Larson from *Rent*)

The older I get, the more I realize I don't want to be around drama, conflict, or stress. I want a cozy home, good food, and to be surrounded by happy people. (Facebook; writer's note—But if my happy people need me, I want to be there for them, stress or not.)

NUTRITION FACT—If you drink a gallon of water per day, you won't have time for other people's drama because you'll be too busy peeing. Stay hydrated, my friends. (Facebook)

It's become increasingly apparent to me that, as I progress further in time, I spend more of it romanticizing or groaning at my own lost past. I've been trying to balance contending with my past to live fully while not falling prey to the whole spilled-milk deal. It's strange how something so unattainably long gone sways us. Anyway, I guess my aging has been a cycle of thinking about such things for an hour or so, then forgetting about it entirely as I get swept away in activities I'll romanticize or groan at later. That and heartburn. (My Darrah-Do, all of age 23)

Y'all, enjoy those twenties, thirties, and forties because, in your fifties, that check engine light gonna come on. (Facebook)

You are never too old to set another goal or to dream new dreams. (C. S. Lewis, writer)

Give your flowers ahead of time. Those $5 bouquets from the grocery store went a long way for seven years with Mother.

Be nice and realize lots of people are dealing with hard issues that don't show on the outside but are presenting a good face to the world. So sometimes just turn the other cheek. All our time on earth will end, so enjoy yourself. Also look and dress your age as you are what you are. [Writer's note—Mary, can we have a talk? See page 73.] Also be glad you live in America. Not that everything is rosy for everybody, but better here than lots of places in the world. Just watch the news! (Mary, age 87)

Words of Wisdom—Life is like a tapestry woven of lumpy, bumpy "fibers"; soft, smooth threads; prickly situations; scratchy times; smooth sailings; sunny bright yellows; and down-in-the-dumps blues. But there will NEVER be another tapestry woven like yours. Mine has a tremendous amount of crazy purple!

Speaking of fabric, *Southern Living* magazine, on May 1, 2020, in an article by Betsy Cribb, has declared "The Housedress Is Officially Back, and We Are Here for It!" Now… what exactly was that housedress that my great, great-aunt used to wear? But NO, *SL* means 100 percent cool cotton muumuus and caftans and maxis giving unrestrictive movement! Sign me up!

Age has allowed me to compliment teens, where I never would have when I was younger. EVERYBODY needs morale boosters. I just hope when I tell the guys they're cuties that they realize I'm the age of their grandmothers. I don't care what people think; I'm meaning it in the nicest of ways. Is that sexual harassment?

There's a fine line between crazy and free spirited, and it's usually a prescription. (Facebook)

Relax…we're all crazy; it's not a competition.

Some people aren't just missing a screw; the whole toolbox is gone. (Facebook)

A true friend is someone who knows how crazy you are and is still willing to be seen in public with you. (Facebook)

What I thought would make me productive:
HARD WORK
What actually does:
LESS THAN HALF WORK +
AN EQUAL AMOUNT OF EXERCISE, HEALTHY EATING, AND SLEEP

AND THE REMAINDER...TIME OFF
(Facebook)

You cannot raise your children the way your parents raised you because your parents raised you for a world that no longer exists.
Children are the rainbow of life.
Grandchildren are the pot of gold.
If I had known how much fun grandchildren would be, I'd have had them FIRST!

Grandchildren don't make a man feel old; it's knowing that he's married to a grandmother. (G. Norman Collie, former Philadelphia and New York City newspaper editor)

The older I get, the more I realize that the things that cost nothing hold the most value. (Facebook)

Oh, have you ever noticed as you age that your nose runs when you eat? Just wait!

Middle Age in a Nutshell

1. "Wait… What did I come in here for?"
2. "I could've SWORN that was my password!"
3. "Sorry, I forgot what I was going to say."
4. "Why is the print to these instructions so *tiny*?"
5. "Who cares if it looks good? I'm comfortable."
6. "Has anyone seen my phone?"
7. "Stupid scale…that *cannot* be right!"
8. "Huh, I wonder how I got this bruise…"
9. "Shoot, did I already take my vitamin?"
10. "$5 for a box of cereal? They raised the price AND shrunk the box…such a racket!"
11. "Software update *again?* I don't like updates."
12. "Who in the world is calling me at 9:30 p.m.?"

We gotta start thinking about the world we'll leave behind for Betty White when we're all gone. (Facebook)

Unfortunately, Betty White passed away December 31, 2021, seventeen days shy of her one hundredth birthday. Guess this proves that we are all actually gonna go at an unpredictable time. *People* magazine for January 10, 2022, had already posted her picture on its cover, celebrating her birthday.

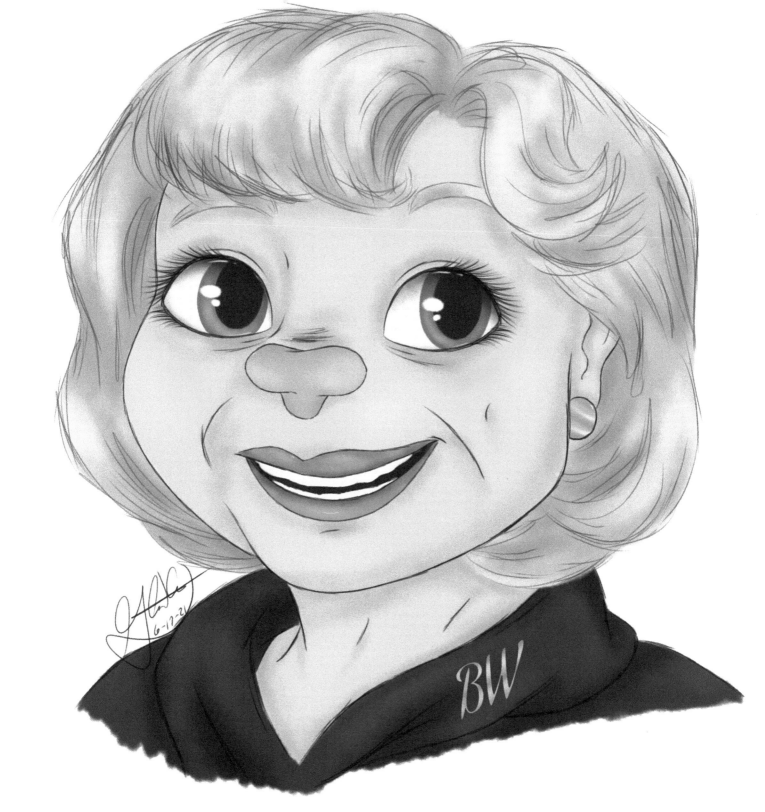

Body, the Nitty-Gritty? Ooey-Gooey? Ukky-Yukky? Achy-Breaky?

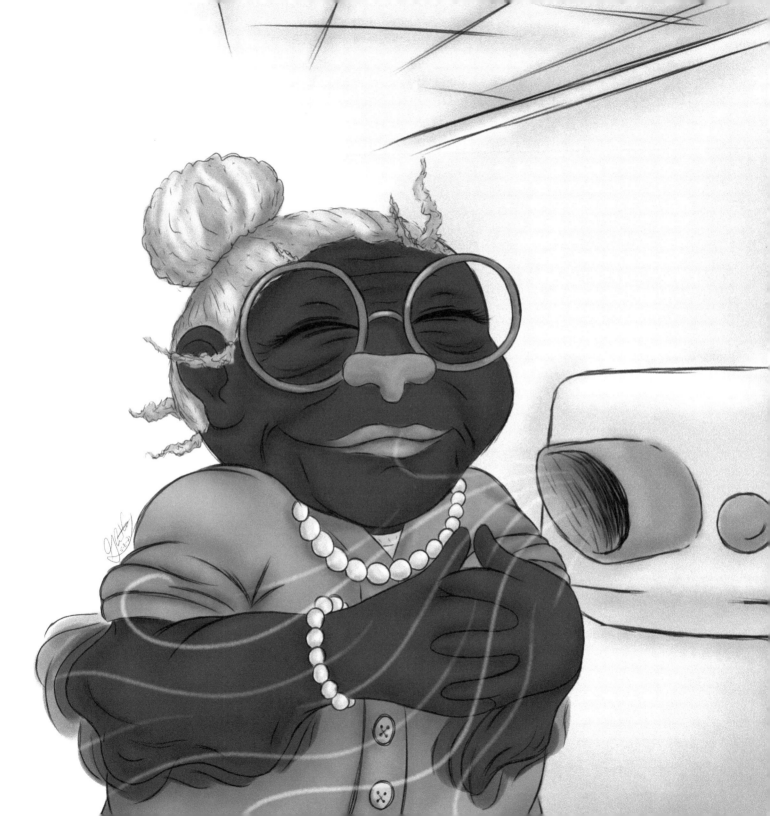

Skin

If they had known the effects of aging, they would have taken better care of their skin. (Becky, Barb, and Peggy, Ocean City, October 2019, ages in the 60s, I think)

Back in the day, baby oil mixed with iodine was the groovy tanning concoction, much like basting a turkey! I didn't use it. But I did start suntanning as SOON as I could tolerate the temps, like late February...in West Virginia...if I stuck flat to the ground to avoid the breeze...and it was really sunny.

What's brown all over and never hides? **SUNSPOTS**, otherwise known as skin cancer teasers. I've found them plentiful on my hands. You may find them on any exposed skin.

The universe must have some kind of vendetta against me because I'm 48 and my FACE IS STILL BREAKING OUT. (Rachel, age 48)

My mother lied to me. My **pimples** did NOT stop at age 20! I'm still waiting! And for my 30th birthday, she gave me MOISTURIZER because it was TIME for it. I was SO insulted! It was hard to argue and impossible for ME to do; but my mother had beautiful skin when she died at 87, as did my grandmother, who had done the same moisturizer thing to my mother. The jury's still out for *moi*.

Vignette

My mother and dad were opposites, who should have never been married to each other. Mother was very naive, prim, and proper to please those around her; but inside, she was a fun-loving girl, like the one playing marbles with the boys in the Norman Rockwell painting. She played piano and organ for the church and everyone who asked her. But her true gift was in accounting. For years, after she quit working for the bank to raise my sister and me, the president would call and ask her to come back with a promise that she'd eventually become a VP.

What the heck do I do with THAT?

With "the aging process" come moles, red spots, white spots, sunspots, pimples, odd bumps, etc. They usually don't mean anything other than—well, the obvious—you're older than you used to be. BUT when in doubt, check it out. Unfortunately most of us do not have easy access to **Dr. Pimple Popper**, but you should be able to make a dermatologist's acquaintance anyway.

Skin tags—well, that's what regular people call them—are just little balls of skin that roll up and bug a person. Mine are on my neck. They're a fine help with necklaces—NOT! IF they're causing a "problem," a dermatologist may remove them. That's usually only covered by insurances if there's a medical problem with them, like pain. This a good time to experience a bout of hypochondria. Back in the "olden" days, people used to tightly tie a thread around them and wait till they turned black and fell off! We didn't mess around in West Virginia!

Watch out for those cute necklaces with the 18-inch chains. They just might disappear under that double chin and strangle you to death. I KNOW you used to wear them, make a shadow box thingy of some kind with them, or donate them.

I'd get out in the wind, and by God, the wind would blow my skin off! (OR, age 90-something) But at that age, he was still "ginsenging" and drinking enough that the sheriff would have to drive him home, and the deputy would drive his car. Fun with life was the secret to his longevity. (Recounted by Kenny, his nephew, age 76)

Vignette

OR (Ollie) was Kenny's uncle, who lived to the ripe age of 99. He attributed that to smoking, hitting the bottle, and ginsenging, which he did all his life, I suppose. Ginsenging consists of climbing our West Virginia hills and pushing through the brush and the brambles, over the rattlesnakes and around the bears, to get this quite valuable root sold largely in Asian markets that's just available certain times of the year. He sold a bit, but I guess it may have been part of his longevity because he kept a root in his pocket and chewed on it all the time. He claimed it was the alcohol that preserved him.

WARNING: Besides finding the way, your skin now flaps in the wind, or from Costco hand dryers, like waving plains of grains (I watched in horror the first and maybe second times), if your natural protective covering drops its guard at all, it will thin and tear like soggy toilet paper. And, God forbid, if you're on blood thinners, you could bleed to death from a paper cut!

Prepare for the general sag of pretty much everything. It's okay. You're getting older; it's supposed to. Now, if you choose to "do something about it," on like your face, even entertainment personalities cannot deny the real story told by their necks and hands.

And in a similar vein, in 2021, there are TONS of lovely tattoos that are going to be, well, NOT lovely when they experience their sag. Think "LLLOOOVVVEEE" and the butterfly from hell that only shows up when you have a colonoscopy! OH, and the sexy breast ones that will slide to your saggy belly button.

For all the young ladies thinking of getting a tattoo, REMEMBER—when you get older, a butterfly on the back becomes a buzzard in the crack. (Facebook; writer's comment—HAHAHAHAHAHAHAHAHA)

An 81-year old woman went in to get her first tattoo. As the tattoo artist worked the needle over the intricate design, she found herself more and more curious, until she couldn't help but ask the woman, "Why are you getting a tattoo this late in life?"

The old woman grinned and replied, "Well, it's something I've wanted to do since my 50s, but I figured if I waited, we could just incorporate the sagging into the design! (*Older Jokes for Older Folks*)

How does a 36C become a 32 long? (Barbara, age 68)

Actually it seems that, after a certain point, breasts' locations and shapes change with each ensuing decade...and may change independently of each other.

There is a story about an older lady who thought she just might commit suicide. Her life had gotten pretty lonely. So she called her doctor to ask where the heart was located. She had it figured that that would be a pretty permanent end if she shot herself there. He carefully explained that it was located between her breasts. Okay.

Several hours later, an older woman showed up in the ER with a gunshot wound to her knee.

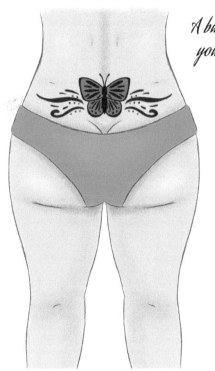

A butterfly on your back...

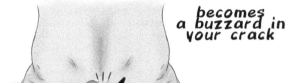

becomes
a buzzard in
your crack

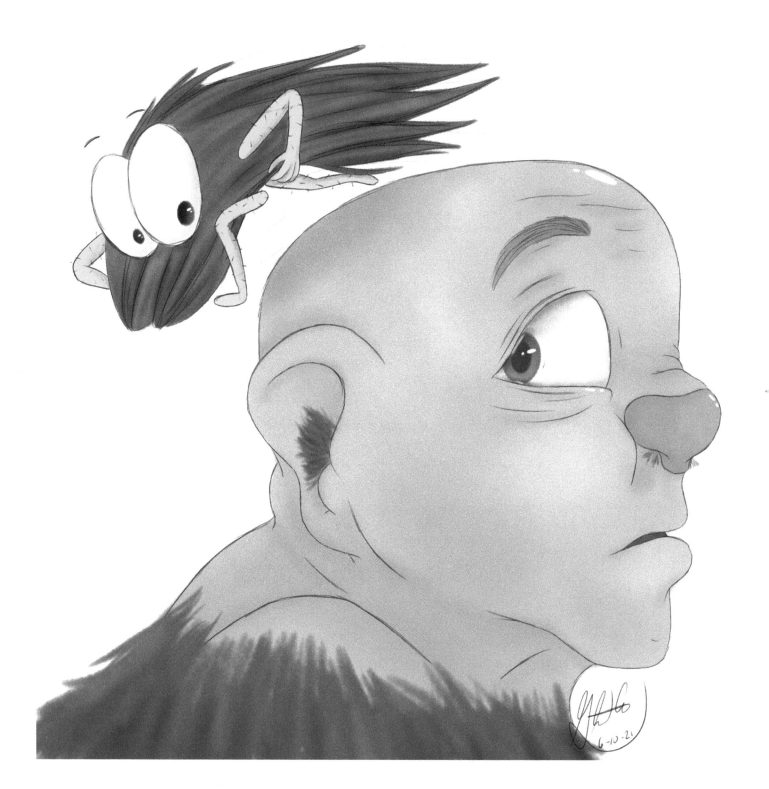

Hair

Hey, where's your wild hair color? I'm disappointed. (Larry, golfer, age 63)

Me, glumly—Gray doesn't hold ANY color! $85 down the drain, literally. I guess purple's out for my birthday. BUT by golly, I tried it…one…more…time for my sixty-seventh birthday! And it's STILL in! After three days…three weeks. Now it's not. Now it's COVID hair—longer, stringer, AND COMING IN, IN A VERY ACCEPTABLE SHADE OF, WELL, GRAY/BLONDISH! And I'm amazed to discover that I can still grow hair! After being sheared short for so long, I thought the days of hair growth were OVER… Now, I can make a MINI ponytail! It may not be pretty, but it makes me happy.

Remember W-A-Y back when the older ladies out in public had blue hair? Wonder where they found that stuff? It covered up THEIR gray, didn't it?

I'm just glad to still have hair. (Pastor Buck, age 69)

In the absence of hair, commonly referred to as baldness, and with thinning hair, do remember to wear a hat ANYTIME the sun exists. That means on sunny days and cloudy days. On rainy days, you're probably safe. If you can't wear a hat for some obscure reason, slather that pate with sunscreen because sun can do some real damage in the form of precancers and cancers, which initially are treated with this icy-cold spray that soon causes some pain and a large bubble, which will eventually dissipate but indicate to the dermatologist that you need regular appointments to potentially do the same repeatedly. Mr. Ayers, a golfer (hint: SUN), has now graduated to blue treatments where they cook his noggin willy-nilly and hit all the potentials at once. No, he's not comfortable after that. God forbid on one of these trips that they'd cook him too deeply and hit empty space.

You know, jokes have been made about male baldness ad infinitum.

> About 60% of men are nearly bald by age 50. 20% of men are bald by
> the age of 30. (Bob Doyle, *Cumberland Times-News*, January 12, 2020)

HOWEVER, female baldness is just not funny, especially if your mother had very thin hair. They even put wood fiber in my mother's to "make it look fuller." My knowledgeable hairstylists told me that perming would hurt my hair. So I stopped. (Hated perms anyway from the time I was 4 when my aunt got hold of me.) Then they told me that, although it would make my hair appear thicker, hair coloring would damage my hair. Being blonde, or peach or burgundy or green for that matter, wouldn't make a difference. After years of experimenting starting with Sun-In in the 60s, I have discovered they may have been right... SO if I stand under a light, my hair looks like the Amazon rainforest after harvest! It's just going, going, gone! However, hair DOES thin as we age. That's my story, and I'm sticking to it! But men aren't the only ones who can become bald!

Morale booster hint for women with thinning hair—Get a little real hair hairpiece and have it shaped to fit your hairstyle and be the same color (not like the cheap—well, not all THAT cheap—one about which my hairdresser children laughed me out of the shop), and nobody will be the wiser! Just make sure you still have enough hair to snap it into! (Source withheld for fear she might excommunicate me.)

As we ladies age, it seems that our hair is cut shorter and shorter. That seems to be the norm. From my position in the choir loft, I could view the aging congregation with their short gray bobs... AWK! Then I was caught up on the very few who have chosen to leave that stuff long and flowing at 60-something (I love you, N, but you know who you are). Choice, I know, and that's all I'm gonna say about that. But wait, I am learning, since my hair has grown during COVID, what it's like to have a ponytail to stick out of the hole in my baseball cap at the beach! I'm feeling at least several decades younger!

However, it's been an eye-opening experience watching people turn gray in the congregation. It's a joke among United Methodists that we all have our chosen seats, and God forbid someone should sit in OUR seat! But it's been very disturbing to see those seats vacate due to aging and death. I'm heartbroken to go past Bill's chosen seat and not be able to knock his elbow off the arm...on my way up to communion...every time. Well, he started it by messing up my hair EVERY time he caught me off-guard! In church! I'm sure God likes for us to laugh!

Why is it that women start losing their hair as they get older, but it starts growing out of their nostrils, and it's long and dark? I thought that was only supposed to happen to men? Or is it just me? And then I have this one wild, curly black hair on my jaw line that I have to pluck every once in a while... I always look for it. But I can never find it till it's about 2 inches long! C'mon, friends of mine! I KNOW you've had to see it! You're supposed to tell me about these things! And it looks like it doesn't belong to anyone in my gene pool! (Jill, age 64; writer's note—Jill and I have both made the SAME certain person close to us PROMISE that, if we become incapacitated for some reason, he will PLUCK those scurrilous under-the-chin beasts! And sadly for him, it is my son who has promised to do that for me...and for his Aunt Jill. HYSTERICAL LAUGHTER!)

(Writer's note: Unfortunately, Jill lost her fight with pancreatic cancer in June 2021, giving her nephew a break from the plucking curse.)

Before we heard of Bill Cosby's fall from grace, he was a great comedian. When he turned 50, he discussed how all the hair from the top of his head had slid down his body to settle in "other" less desirable places. This could explain why men grow hair IN THEIR EARS! Who knew? I think mine ended up under my chin along with my leg hair that disappeared. Just sayin'.

My dad died at 84 with a beautiful shock of thick white hair. My mother had nice, hard teeth all her life. What did I end up with? My dad's soft teeth and my mother's thin hair. Genetics cannot be denied, Jill!

Vignette

My dad appears several times in this book. He was quite a character in most ways for 80 or so years and was usually out of sorts and mean, especially when aggravated by alcohol. During the 75th anniversary of WWII, I found that alcohol was the comforter for many of those soldiers who tried to forget what they'd seen and done. I always felt that there was a nicer person in him, but he kept it well hidden. Mother and I finally deduced that he may have been learning disabled or had Asperger's because he always thought he was right and the world did things backward. I DREADED the thought of trying to get him to the nursing home when his dementia became more than Mother could handle. But I asked him to go take a look...and he settled in! He sang songs at the top of his voice with the others using ANY words that came out of his mouth; one day, he covered up the lady parked outside his door each day who said over and over that she was cold and almost got himself kicked out! He'd put the blanket over her head! But most importantly, for the remaining 18 months of his life, he became a funny, carefree spirit who finally told me he loved me and became my DADDY!

Age mellows some people; others it makes rotten. (*Old Jokes for Old Folks*)

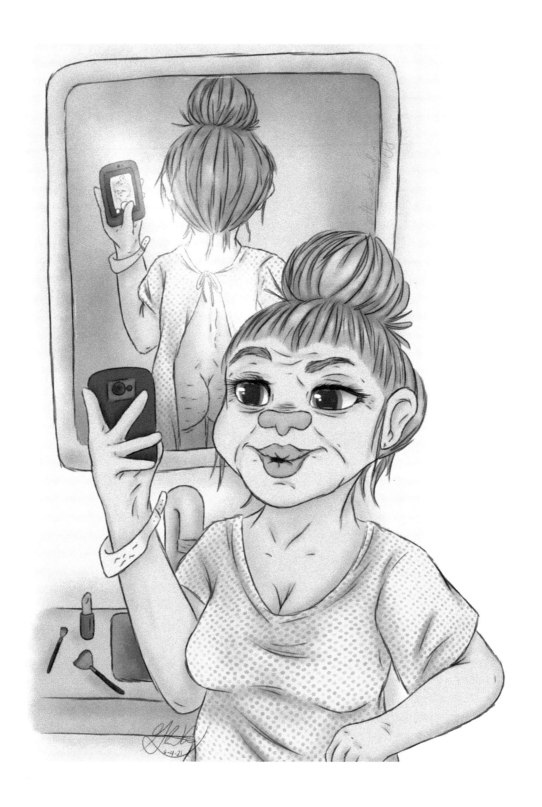

Wrinkles and Other Such Things

Bags and wrinkles go together! Knees, boobs, chin, neck, ears, arms, and butt.

In the near future, little old ladies won't be able to knit, sew, or quilt; but they'll take awesome self-pics in the bathroom mirror...wrinkles and all! (Facebook)

I think my body is competitive... My face and boobs are having a race as to which one can slide and hang faster!
And if I have "wings" now, why can't I fly?
Who are you? Yes, the memory is a nuisance now too." (Dear cousin Kelly, age 59)

Question—Is it okay, as a late 70s or 80s-ish person in Florida, to go into a convenience store in a bikini with your old, wrinkly butt cheeks bagging out without adequate coverage?
Answer—After some deliberation and in consideration that there was a towel clasped to her sagging bazooms, I decided that, if she had the courage to do it, I had the courage to accept it. Then I saw the sports car in which her aged husband waited for her, and I just threw up my hands and thought, *What the heck!* I'll get used to it, I think. But for now, I'm just concentrating on getting my hands away from being firmly planted over my disbelieving open mouth and yearning to have that bravery at that age! But... I am forever changed.

HOWEVER, should you discover one side of your face bagging suddenly, like our friend Rene's did upon awakening, don't panic; but with expediency, get yourself checked for (a) stroke (discussed later under the "Body Proper") or (b) Bell's palsy.

Symptoms (limited to one side of your face) of <u>Bell's palsy</u>:
— Inability to close eyelid or blink
— Eye waters more or less than usual
— Difficulty chewing
— Decreased sense of taste
— Facial muscles twitch
— Pain or numbness behind the ear
Most people recover completely within 3 months. (WebMD)

OMIGOSH! I FINALLY HAVE A CLEAVAGE...AND IT'S WRINKLING INSTEAD OF CLEAVING!
But you could go braless; it'll pull the wrinkles out of your face.
Here's a clothing dilemma only understood by LARGE-busted women. This was over-heard in the clothing section of a delightful Myrtle Beach department store.

> (*Whisper, whisper.*) I have to be so careful what I wear because my
> bra straps cut into my shoulders!

Now I know this one for a fact because, during my short but fateful waitressing gig (I actually poured salad dressing down a guy's back; thank God he was a preacher!), I made the acquaintance of a large-busted older server who, from years of being on her feet and carrying heavy trays, had literally a crevasse I could lay my finger in! Wonder why she complained about her shoulders aching?

Some bras, 50 (?) years later, now have wider padded straps, which may help. Or there's the route of breast reduction, which several relatives have taken. BUT for crying out loud, **never** consider going without one in public. That can be just a jiggly, fat, ugly mess from which children's eyes must be shielded! And you will find them in a M-U-C-H lower location—the boobs, I mean.

When I was younger, I could hook, unhook, and take my bra off at will (as could some guys, if I wasn't growling loudly enough!). Now hooking is a challenge ending in a dead sweat willing those 2 ends to meet. NO, I will not go up another size!

And God forbid you should try to pull a tankini swimsuit with a built-in bra over your head during the sticky summer! They roll up like rubber bands under your armpits, and there you stand helpless with your boobs strangling half in and half out. And nothing you try will allow you to reach that confound thing to unwrap it! After struggling for 15 minutes one day, I thought I was going to have to put on a shirt and go to the beach that way to get help! Then God provided me with one little scrap of fabric which I could use to pull it down. Whew!

Speaking of breasts / bazooms/ the girls / Tatas or—as breast cancer groups sometimes boldly put it—boobies, get those rascals **mammogramed** annually or as often as your GYN advises for your age group. Sure, being clamped between 2 cold metal plates is anything but thrilling, but it beats the alternative, if there should be a problem! And yes, men can get breast cancer also. Get lumps checked ASAP!

I had a second set of holes poked in my ears when I got real diamond earrings because I felt sure I'd lose them if they weren't attached to me, and I tightened the screw backs faithfully. However, in my mid-60s, I began to lose a diamond here and a diamond there, which was astounding considering the back was still attached to the darned thing when I found it! When it happened a third time and it precipitated a complete search of the church grounds after candlelight service, I decided to study on the situation a little more closely. What to my wondering eyes should appear but that my ears WERE SAGGING TOO! The weight of the bottom earring was pulling down the hole of my second and diamond earring, and the daggoned thing was popping out slick as a whistle! I don't wear them anymore lest I should need a stitch to tighten the hole! BTW, the lost jewel showed up at home. I forgot it fell out before we left for our trip. They are stored in 2 separate places because I found them at 2 different times; I'm afraid that, if I move them, I'll forget where I put them!

As one gauges one's ears with larger and larger holes (ear piercing to the extreme), consider the effects of aging and exactly where you'd like to find that sagging, thinning skin. In your grandbaby's hands and being used as a teething ring? Clipped up and around to frame your professional appearance? Lying on your shirt collar for the church directory picture when you're in your 70s? Stop laughing. You're probably not that far-off now!

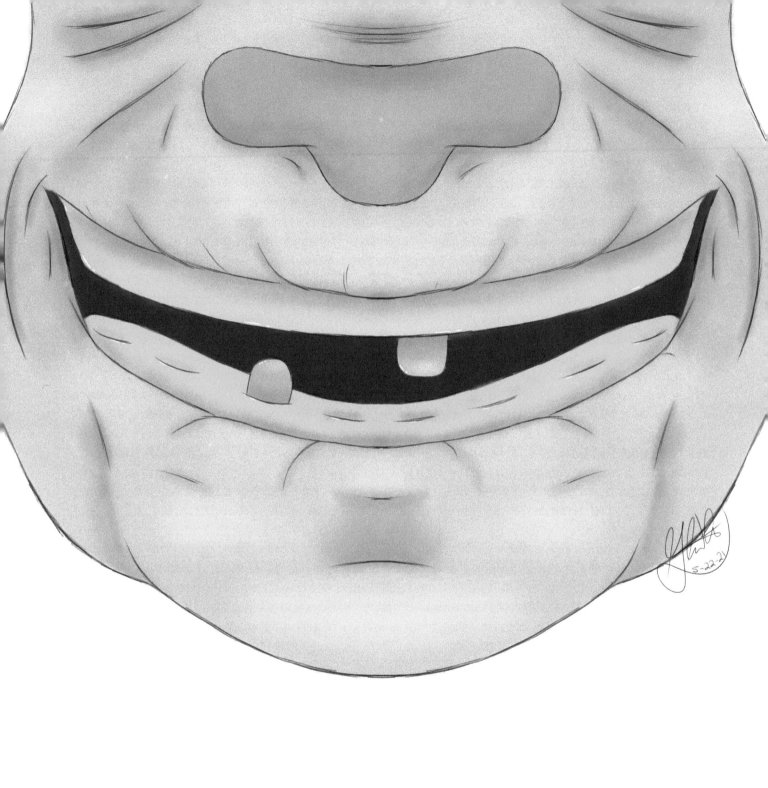

Mouth

Eat what you want while you still have teeth! (Plaque in a dentist's office)

Aging brings a whole lot of problems for your mouth. After all, some of those teeth have been in there HOW long, and you've exposed them to HOW many sodas and sweets and HOW much crunchy or sticky stuff and opened HOW many packages of foods, etc. There are crowns, bridges, root canals (a very primitive process in my book!), and implants, to name a few methods of correcting problems. So unless you want to look like a Toothless Wonder, you will probably be familiarizing yourself with these. Therefore, the term *golden years* actually refers to the gold per dollar put into this area and several others, not what you were misled to believe. Sorry, Drs. Tim.

> Bridges and crowns are all MINE, because they're connected to my body, and I paid for them! (Diana, retired music teacher, age 72)

Question—To electric toothbrush or to not electric toothbrush?
Answer—It may depend on how well your wrist and hand work. Arthritis, for one, can be a bear affecting your decision.
Question—To repair or to replace your teeth?
Answer—See above about Toothless Wonder.

And to those who wear lipstick, DO be aware that lipstick does creep and crawl into those lines forming around your mouth. Time to look for a product that DOES NOT MOVE once it's on your lips, and keep in mind that your potentially shakier hands are going to provide a real challenge to your accuracy. Once it's on, wherever it lands, it DOES NOT MOVE! I have found, however it lands, that that touch of color gives my whole face and, therefore, demeanor a lift. Thank you, Kathy P., for setting the example and helping in one more way.

Kenny says he can't smell, but he can taste. How is that possible?

Oh, with enough age, taste and smell may be impaired. But, KENNY, how is THAT possible?

Brooke Shields, actress, age 55 reveals on a recent Colgate ad that she looks forward to seeing what's next in her life but not gum disease. OH NO...one more unrealized thing.

However, loss of taste and smell can also be COVID related rather than age related. We now know.

As one ages, the voice lowers. Change rows in the choir!

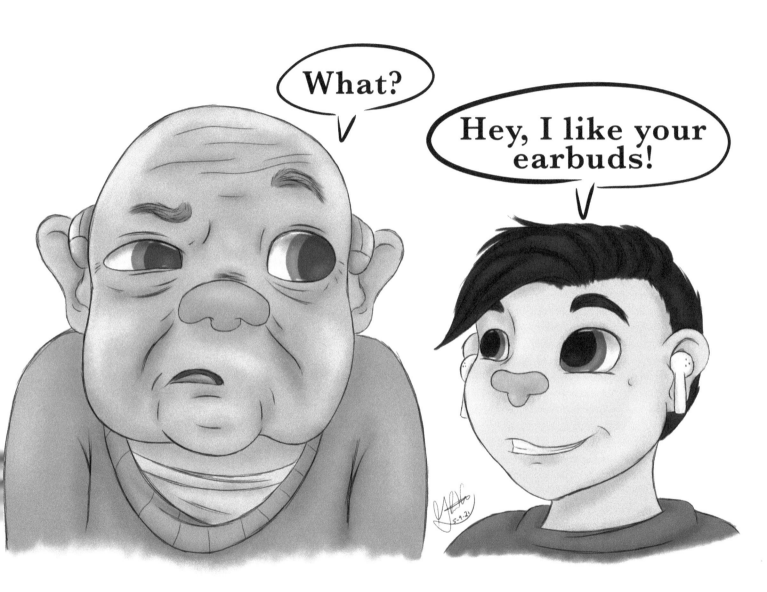

Ears

An elderly couple was attending church services. About halfway through the sermon, the husband leaned over and said, "I just let out a silent fart. What do you think I should do?"

The wife replied, "Put a new battery in your hearing aid." (*Old Jokes for Old Folks*; writer's note—BWAHAHAHAHAHAHA!)

Vignette

Kenny is my husband and confidant on all my crazies, bless his heart. Sometimes he gets it; sometimes he has a deer-in-the-headlights look. I tossed him into his 70s W-A-Y ahead of me so I could see what happens. Heck, nobody believes his age. He golfs, mows the grass, does kitchen stuff, and takes care of me. I'm the one who gives the 70s a bad name. And I'm not even there yet! He says he's my "butler"; I say, "Sometimes, he's the butt!"

Me: Kenny...KENNY...**KENNY**!
Him, growling: I HEARD you! You don't have to YELL!
Me, having had a full conversation with no response from him: Did you hear me?
Him—No response either!

Hearing deteriorates in most people as they age. The speed at which it goes is largely determined by exposure to loud sounds in the workplace, equipment around the house, accidents, and—I predict, in the future—the use of earphones, and more. It is not a sign of aging or damage of pride to have a hearing exam. It's smart. That will merely show you the level of sounds you might miss. And it's for your own safety. However, if you're missing a large range of sounds indicated by turning the TV up louder, inability to distinguish conversations in a room full of people, driving your spouse freaking crazy, and alienating people because you're not responding or not responding appropriately, it's probably time to be checked for hearing aids. There are some very good ones on the market now that screen out much of the environmental sounds that used to bug wearers. And you'll be surprised at what you've been missing. Be aware that untreated hearing loss can lead to difficulties with significant others, isolation, problems negotiating various environments, loss of mental functioning, and earlier dementia.

Also, consider hearing loss services as you tend to your older relatives' needs or think about moving your parents. In an AP article in the *Hampshire Review*, Romney, West Virginia, on April 28, 2021, this importance is discussed as a part of what is referred to as late-deafness needs being addressed by Mary Ann Vividen's Eastern Panhandle Deaf Alliances Inc. During the pandemic, the use of technology—in particular Wavello, a video call system—helped people stay connected regardless of hearing function, thus decreasing some of the isolation. People who are late-deaf are in a unique situation though, because, most of the time, they are not sign users; and my experience is that they are not inclined to learn a new communication system like that. However, as technology becomes more available, it may be more successful at keeping these individuals in the loop.

Persons with COCHCLEAR IMPLANTs due to hearing loss have more susceptibility to pneumonia and should be extra cautious to not be exposed. If you wonder what the cochlear implant looks like, look at pictures of Rush Limbaugh. His was quite visible on the side of his head behind his ear.

Another hearing loss phenomenon hit Huey Lewis in the 80s and virtually ended his career for nearly 40 years. Remember him and his '80s group, **Huey Lewis and the News**, and songs like "The Power of Love"? Of course, you do. Turn on your rewind! Well, he was taken down by **Meniere's disease**, a chronic inner ear disorder that causes vertigo and fluctuating hearing loss. He does pretty well hearing speech with his hearing aids, but finding pitch in music is nearly impossible. ("Losing the Sound of Music," *People* magazine, February 17, 2020)

Symptoms of Meniere's disease are sudden attacks of vertigo, tinnitus (a ringing, buzzing, roaring in their ears), hearing loss, and a feeling of fullness in the affected ear. (WebMD)

I randomly met a lovely couple one evening at dinner. We had a delightful exchange. Later I realized how fortunate this lady is. His losing hearing will not be an issue or make her nuts. HE'S DEAF, like possibly born deaf! He was such a funny and friendly guy. (Yes, I sign a smidge to converse a bit...if the receiver is patient enough.)

Speaking of ears, evidently, when I was a child, mine may have stuck out, well, a bit much. Dad referred to them as my "barn doors." Anyway, time and age corrected the problem enough that long hair covered the issue. HOWEVER, with the advent of our life-saving COVID masks with ear straps, I have rediscovered my "barn doors" now sagging and pulled straight out like wings on a plane. No. That is not funny. I need an ear tuck!

Me: Kenny...KENNY...**KENNY**!
Him, growling: WHAT?
Me: DO YOU HAVE YOUR HEARING AIDS ON?
Him, sheepishly: No...
Me, later: KENNY.
Him, with hearing aids on (they're so invisible they're barely noticeable):
    Quit yelling!
(Well, that's a little overkill, but he hears me with the hearing aids on.
That's all that matters, and I believe his golfing buddies would agree!)

Admit it—life would be BORING without me!

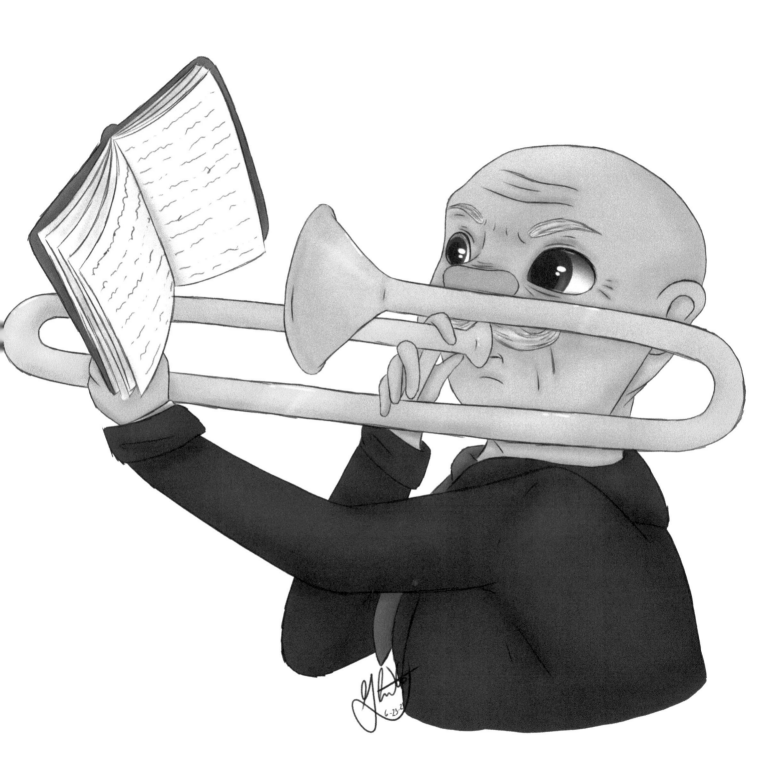

Eyes

Yesterday I stumbled, again, over a concrete car bumper. And I finally figured out part of the reason that uneven surfaces, odd or unexpected steps, irregularities in pavement, etc. are a problem. I don't see them! With bifocals for reading (close vision), when I look down, the vision is distorted because I'm not reading. Decreasing night vision (the ability to see clearly at night / drive a car at night) also contributes to more likelihood of falling. Aging…HARUMPH! (This also goes with falls, page 61.)

> You know you're getting old when "Friends with Benefits" means having someone who can drive at night. (Facebook)

Do you know what it's like to be blind or deaf? Well, I predict, based upon my education in blindness and deafness, that a whole new batch of people will become visually impaired and hearing impaired or deaf at earlier ages due to constant <u>screen and earphone use.</u> Sound is being directly sent into the ear canal and is usually amplified. The little cilia/hairs that carry sound are being vibrated more quickly at a closer range and will break off earlier than with normal aging, leading to impaired hearing sooner in life. That's my theory. Screen use exposes the eyes to eyestrain, odd lighting situations, and more wear and tear than one would usually experience. These things shouldn't cause blindness, but eye problems could show up. That's my theory, and it's starting to play out in research.

> (Writer's note—As defined by *Wikipedia*, an <u>optician</u> is the technical practitioner who designs, fits, and dispenses lenses for correction of a person's vision. <u>Optometrists</u> are basic eye-care specialists who can examine, diagnose, and medically treat eye conditions. An <u>ophthalmologist</u> is a type of medical doctor who specializes in surgeries of the eye.)

If... See an...:

1. You have double vision—Optician
2. You see floaters or flashes—Ophthalmologist
3. Your eyes feel dry—Optician
4. You have a sharp pain in your eye—Ophthalmologist
5. Your vision is unusually blurry—Ophthalmologist
6. You're losing peripheral (side vision) vision—Ophthalmologist
7. You're having trouble reading—Optometrist
8. You see dark spots in the center of your vision—Ophthalmologist
9. You have reduced night vision—Optometrist
10. You see glare when you drive—Ophthalmologist

(Jessica Magala, "How to Treat the 10 Top Vision Problems," **AARP**, January 30, 2020)

Funny thing about getting older—your eyesight may weaken, yet you can see through people much better. (Facebook)

After you turn 50 years old, you can't recognize letters close, but you can recognize idiots from far away. (Facebook)

Cataracts—Should your vision become steadily more and more, well, foggy, colors are not as bright as you thought they should be, and it's harder to see clearly, panic not. It could well be a cataract(s). Now, when you see the doctor, he will probably tell you you're not going blind. But he may tell you that you do have a **cataract**; and IF you haven't been seeing your eye doctor annually like you really should, that rascal may already be "ripe," which is doctorese for "You need to get on my surgery schedule." Your cornea has become occluded, usually WITH AGE, and needs to be replaced. As I understand it (mine isn't ripe yet) from friends who have already taken the big step, it's not that big a deal. And before you panic, take comfort in knowing that this surgery has taken huge strides in postsurgery practices. You will need someone to take you home, and you cannot lift anything remotely heavy for ten days or so or bend more than waist level. THEN you're on with your life!

Macular degeneration—If the doctor tells you this, you may pale a little because it occurs largely in older folks. With this one, central vision will decrease till only peripheral or side vision remains. It will make recognizing people's faces and reading difficult, BUT you are not totally blind. It is what it is. Ask people in your environment to not move things around but to remove fall hazards. This will help you find things and avoid things. Oh, and you will eventually not be able to drive.

> According to my source who has it, "It is hereditary." (Jean, age 88; writer's note—who knew?)

Vignette

Ila has been a sweetheart of the community for ninety years. Although she spent most of those years in the funeral home—okay, in the house above the funeral home where her family's funeral business was located—she was mostly known for her musical involvement. She sang in various groups for a variety of shows, but she played the piano or organ for EVERYTHING! For example, she sang in the choir and played the organ for church for at least 70 years. She also gathered everyone around her piano for sing-alongs for all the holidays, played and sang at the nursing homes, and played for funerals as needed. When her macular degeneration showed up and she could no longer read the notes or the words, she managed to fool most of us for a long time because her huge repertoire of memorized music allowed her to keep right on playing.

> I get mad at myself for forgetting things ("which leads to tears that never happened before," added her grandson Nicholas, age 40). I've lost my eyesight, and now I'm losing my hearing! (Ila, age 92)

According to Nicholas, she's experiencing extreme frustration; however, she can play hymns/songs for 2 hours at a time from memory, once a month, at a senior center she visits.

When you are frustrated with me because of the things I cannot do...just imagine how frustrated I must be because I'm no longer able to. (Facebook)

Light floors make things more visible as you age. (Kathy, Kay, and Diana, ages 84, 74, and 72)

Yes, and don't move things around in a living area for a visually declining person! Like, don't get all excited about "cleaning up" for your elderly uncle because he will inevitably take a nosedive over something you've moved "to help him out." We humans memorize our patterns, especially in traveling through our houses in the dark, etc. Don't move the rugs, the dogs, and the junk because chances are the visually declining person knows how to steer around the critters to get to the TV remote.

Do be aware that there may be services available to people with declining vision that may help them negotiate their environment even outside their houses. For example, in the same AP article from the *Hampshire Review*, Romney, West Virginia, April 28, 2021, that was mentioned for late-deafened services, Tina Burns, the director of resource development for the Shenandoah Community Health Foundation providing these, mentioned the importance of vision monitoring, because "10% of their patients in 2020 had diabetes" and many of those patients didn't receive screenings appropriate for the disease. Monitoring the eyes is as necessary as that of other major organs affected by diabetes. After a certain age, people may start to notice that their arms are just not quite long enough anymore. No matter how far they stretch them to hold their reading materials, they still cannot quite see that print clearly! It's a musical problem called trombone vision.

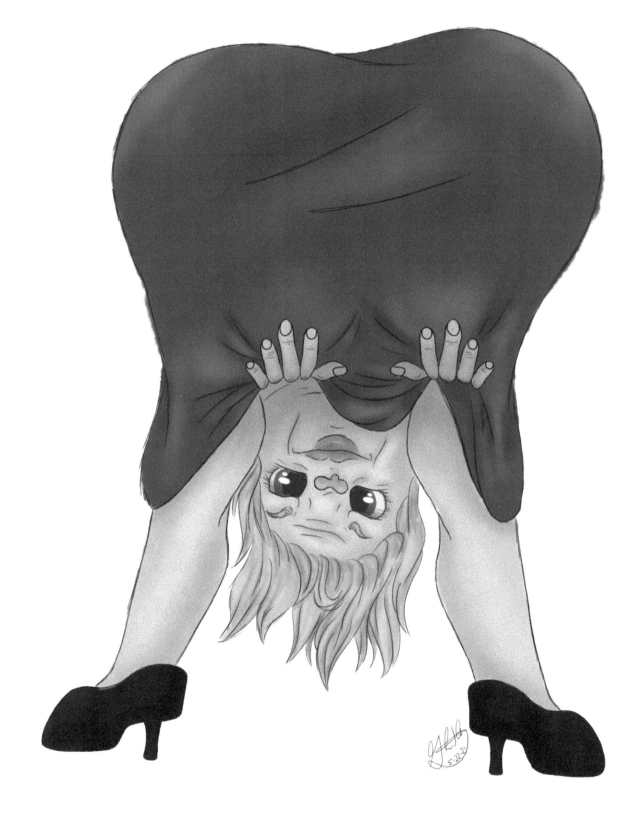

Legs, Feet, and Hands

History of the aging shoe-addicted wearer:

Youthhood somewhere—"Oooo, goodie, my first pair of heels!"

Beginning workday world—"Let's try these 4 inch spikes."

Middle work years—"My feet are killing me! I can't wait to get home and get out of these shoes!"

Retirement—"If I have to wear old flat granny shoes, they'd better have CHARACTER!"

Be prepared that, if you sit in any odd position for a period of time, you WILL have to retrain your legs when you stand and utter that forever-used phrase "OH!" or just grunt. I feel sure this is where it originated.

> You don't really realize how old you are until you sit on the floor and then try to get back up. (Facebook)

> When I hit 40, it was like the "check engine" light came on! I couldn't get off the floor after wrapping presents! (Diana, nurse practitioner, age 42)

And for heaven's sake, don't sit on the floor unless you have a battle plan for getting up! Or maybe a task analysis involving which foot or knee you can still use well enough with the hand that better by darned have a STRONG grip on the sturdiest thing in the room! I don't know about others, but though I appreciate a proffered hand of help for getting up, said hand does nothing for the above task analysis and may actually send you spinning sideways and upsot! Or worse yet, send both of you ass-over-teacup in a pile on the floor. Getting up in an A-frame position with your butt in the air is still preferable to either of those.

Fingers begin to not respond to the command of "tie my shoes," etc.! They think it's funny that I'm seeing what they should do and they're just playing around!

> After a while, you just cannot trust using only one hand; pick up stuff
> with two hands. (Diana, age 72)

Hands get stiff. That means that they're just not working as they did when you were 20. Playing the piano and organ are more challenging for Diana. Opening jars may require a stronger set of hands or, to maintain your independence, a rubber jar opener, a fancy but relatively simple device meant for aging hands that can be found on the internet under assistive devices; or jar openers; or a table knife to pound those infuriating edges that won't give until the seal releases. Don't you feel better now?

Note to manufacturers of stuff like shampoo, bath products, back brushes, and other such products, please put on some stiff gloves with Vaseline on them and try to open your cotton-picking products before you try to market them. Not very efficient in a lot of cases, huh? And not a darned bit funny either!

Also, fingers may become larger due to arthritis or weight gain (yes, I said it), thereby requiring resizing of rings. Either resize them or stop wearing them. Do not let vanity cause you to visit the ER to get them cut off when your hands swell!

Heed this red flag warning: Ocean surf that you USED to love wading in will, at a certain age or balance or fear of falling, easily flip your butt right down in that slurpy stuff, going back out and fill the seat of your swimsuit with sand. You'll be digging that stuff out of crevices you never knew you had for DAYS! But do not despair; save your quarters—well, bills and other change also—and purchase a handy-dandy, STURDY, short (but not TOO short) beach chair, which you can plunk right in that surf, sit yourself down, have your feet in the water, and read your *People* magazine knowing you are not going to fall. Just take note of whether you're in high or low tide. High tide currently means moving chair toward the water as it recedes. Low tide means to not become absorbed in your magazine and forget that the tide is moving in and will eventually submerge you, the chair, *People*, and all if you do not frequently move yourself farther up the beach, especially if you have balance issues. However, before you commit to sitting there, be sure to develop a plan for getting out of said chair. You're on your own on that one! I personally scoot out of the chair onto my knees, turn around, and use the chair arms to steady myself. It might not be pretty, but neither is being flat out in the sand...or slurp! Also keep in mind that that lovely surf will bury the legs of your chair in the wet sand...and play tug with you. Just sayin'.

OMIGOODNESS! I decided to play one of those ridiculous game thingies on Facebook to see what they predicted I might look like when I'm 97. Well...much to my wondering eyes appeared an old lady bent over, grabbing her ankles and looking at me between her legs! Now this might be completely wrong for most people; however, my real picture that they'd used to determine this showed me with flaming plum-colored hair tied in a bandana 1940s style. 'Nuff said?

Advice—Do NOT let the podiatrist be the one to find a second set of socks and 3 toe pads in the toes of the shoes you've just worn into his office. Okay, so I was in a hurry when I put them on! And I'm aging. And I have neuropathy. Oh...be aware that you could find yourself asking him, "You're gonna carve **WHAT** off my toe? (In many cases, review "diabetes.")

Question: Do you think that, when we die, they'll have to pry our cellphones from our cold, hard fingers? And that our fingers will stay in that grip position as the earth falls in on us, or fire consumes us, or what-ever your choice? Omigosh, the funeral directors might have to break them (mortuary secret) to prepare your beautiful presentation for your friends and family!

Question: If someone from the 1950s suddenly appeared, what would be the most difficult thing to explain to them about life today?

Answer: I possess a device in my pocket that is capable of accessing the entirety of information known to man. I use it to look at pictures of cats and get into arguments with strangers. (Facebook)

The Body Proper

When you're over 40 and they say, "Just put a Band-Aid where it hurts…"

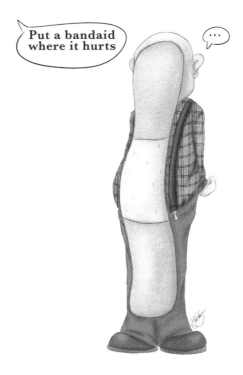

After 30, a body has a mind of its own. (Bette Midler, American actress)

Welcome to middle age. No one tells you that rigor mortis starts while you're still alive. (Facebook)

Every morning, I wake up in Spain...the S is silent. (Facebook)

I really don't mind getting older, but my body is taking it badly. (Facebook)

I went to an antique show...and people were bidding on ME! (Facebook)

Some people try to turn back their odometers. Not me. I want people to know why I look this way. I've travelled a long way, and some of the roads weren't paved. (Facebook)

As I write, it is spring/summer/fall/spring 2020 and 2021 (so I didn't write in winter), and the coronavirus is terrorizing the world. Statistics for the various age groups are still coming in. However, as a rule, older folks and children are more affected by regular flus than are the other age groups. Despite a second round of flu viruses that surged in late January 2020, according to the US Centers for Disease Control and Prevention, "They aren't considered as dangerous to retirement-age [writer's note—nicely put] people." Good news, since most flu deaths and hospitalizations each winter occur in the elderly. In fact, the overall death and hospitalization rates this season are not high "because we haven't seen the elderly as involved in this flu season," said the CDC's Lynnette Brammer.

Amid coronavirus fears, a second wave of flu hits children in the US. (Mike Stobbe, AP medical writer, *Cumberland Times-News*, February 15, 2020; writer's note—This article immediately preceded the influx of COVID the next month, and although COVID devastated our population, this discovery may have led to fewer dual diagnosis cases.)

Perhaps these stats reflect a big push by medical persons and pharmacies for people to get both the flu and pneumonia vaccines. Even my syringe-flinching husband was strapped down at the doctor's office and given both shots. Well, not actually strapped down, but it was a great visual for what nearly happened. As presented today by Vanessa Hochard, RN, age 35, to a church full of white-haired congregants, it is mega important for everyone over 65 to receive the pneumonia vaccine in addition to the flu vaccine. In fact, there are actually 2 types that can protect one from a total of thirty-six of the ninety known pneumonia bacteria. So far, that's as good as it gets, folks; but if we are not protected, the statistics will be worse. In fact, anyone with a compromised immune system, like diabetes or kidney or heart disease, or persons with COPD may receive the vaccines if they are over nineteen and meet specified criteria.

The arrival of COVID vaccines in early 2021 has helped to reduce the devastation of the virus; and all 3—COVID, flu, and pneumonia—are recommended by the CDC.

During flu season and The Time of COVID, follow these guidelines:

1. Wash your hands thoroughly. This is the time it takes to sing the ABC song—in your head.
2. Clean frequently touched surfaces. (Have you noticed that many stores offer disinfectant wipes for use on the cart handles? Take advantage of them! They're free!)
3. "Catch your cough" since bacteria travel through the air when you hack. Even with your hands full, you can always cough into your shoulder/sleeve.

COVID home test kits with rapid turnaround are available as of spring 2021.

> (A kid was standing outside a concert venue that says "THE ARENA—Tonight—'60s Rock 'n' Roll Band," along with some men with walkers and canes.)
> Kid to guys: Aren't you a little old to be listening to a rock and roll band?
> Guys: We ARE the band.

Despite the fact that our beloved '60s and '70s music is still being played 50 years later—WAIT, FIFTY YEARS LATER? It CAN'T have been that long! I'm just figuring out who

I am! That would make somebody pretty old, wouldn't it? ANYWAY, despite the music still sounding the same, baby boomers should dance only in the privacy of their own homes. Our body parts are just not where they used to be, for one thing. Plus women in white socks, tennis shoes, pedal pushers (capris, only baggier), and matronly tops just do not present the same picture as 50 years ago. It's not a pretty one. Even the drop-dead gorgeous hunks are not keeping rhythm with those beer guts. So keep it all at home, how 'bout? I think we're no longer in the Age of Aquarius...

Vignette

Omigoodness! The Age of Aquarius! Even now, I can feel the excitement of that era! Although we weren't in San Francisco or New York, the Age touched us somehow. In Spring 1970 at a small high school in West Virginia that now no longer exists, the junior prom committee was hard at work creating our version of the magical time. 7 great huge honeycomb balls in luscious colors to represent the planets were borrowed from the premier shoe store in the area—almost directly from their display with the warning "Do Not Mess These Up!" Who would, since they came from this prestigious and honored business where their displays made my mouth water? It was like going to a shoe museum to me! Oh, I digress. We hung those fabulous balls from the gym ceiling (don't ask me how because I don't remember) right over a fountain which, in retrospect, seems like a pretty risky plan. And NO, THEY DID NOT GET WET! I don't remember much else about that prom, but it was magical. And I still salivate over shoes...and the **Fifth Dimension**'s "Aquarius / Let the Sunshine In."

So okay, dance in public like nobody's watching. But at least be careful with the clothing BECAUSE people WILL be watching. What else can a lot of them do...other than gossip about things they see?

> I have reached the age where my mind says, "I can do that." But my body says, "Try it and die, fat girl." (Facebook)

I believe this is what happened at the beach when I tore my rotator cuff. Don't ask... I used to do it! But who knew that tailgate was SO high.

Energy drinks increase stroke risk by 500% as irregular heartbeats soar. (From the British Soft Drinks Association, Abigail O'Leary, *Daily Mirror*, December 17, 2018)

Although younger people may be bigger users of these, there are certainly sleep-deprived parents, older adults pushing their bodies for more extra miles, and others trying to survive the general crush of life who might find themselves grabbing an energy drink... because it sounds like a great idea, right? Please be aware just in case. Oh, and kids have strokes too.

Warning signs of a **stroke** (from **WebMD**):

FAST test for strokes—This is used as a quick check for a suspected stroke in yourself or others.
— **F**ace: Smile and see if one side of the face droops.
— **A**rms: Raise both arms. Does one arm drop down?
— **S**peech: Say a short phrase and check for slurred or strange speech.
— **T**ime: If the answer to any of these is yes, call 911 right away and write down the time when symptoms started.

Signs of a **Heart Attack** (from **WebMD**):
— Chest pain
— Shortness of breath
— Dizziness
— Faintness
— Nausea

However, it may feel like a giant fist squeezing the heart or heartburn. Pain may be constant or intermittent. Women may feel symptoms more like jaw, arm, neck, or back pain or a fullness in the chest.

WHEN IN QUESTION, FIND OUT! Don't wait. I tried to convince my husband that he had heartburn at 3:00 a.m., but after writing the check for the paper man and putting it out, he insisted on going to the ER. He was immediately given a clot buster because he was **in the middle of a heart attack.** My mumbling in the night and his sudden concern about the paper could have led to his Waterloo!

According to the **American Heart Association**, in 2008, 356,461 people died in the United States after a sudden cardiac arrest. The heart association reports that more people are surviving sudden cardiac arrest because of increased training and public access to **AEDs** (automated external defibrillator—lightweight, portable devices that deliver an electric shock through the chest to the heart; the shock can potentially stop an irregular heartbeat and allow a normal rhythm to resume following a sudden cardiac arrest— **https://www.heart.org**).

Rates of survival have increased over the last decade because of increased layperson training and public access to AEDs at malls, sporting events, public buildings, and schools, "also corporate and government offices, restaurants and public transport" ("Automated External Defibrillator," *Wikipedia*).

> SPECTATORS: Resuscitation was a Group Effort. (*Cumberland Times-News*, January 26, 2020, page 3A)

Oh, yeah, and the reason for this article was that the spectators and staff at a local high school wrestling match performed this save on a grandfather in the crowd in January 2020.

In the letters to the editor of the *Cumberland Times-News*, Cumberland, Maryland, on September 19, 2020, was a thank you from the very fellow whose life was saved.

> The gratitude and thankfulness I feel is never ending. Please allow me to take this opportunity to offer a heartfelt "thank you" to all the folks in the stands, school faculty, coaching and training staff, EMS, and fire and rescue personnel that made an amazing difference in my life. My heart went into cardiac arrest and needed to be shocked back into rhythm. Since the school has an AED (automated external defibrillator) and personnel trained in its operation, I was able to make a full recovery. Had I been at home, that wouldn't have happened. You are my heroes! (Paul)

Okay, say you're not trained to use an AED; but someone falls to the floor, grabs his/her chest, and stops breathing. You see an AED box on the wall. Yeah, they're clearly labeled. Don't just stand there waiting for some trained individual to show up and watching the poor soul die. Yell for someone to call 911. Then grab that box, open it, and listen to the directions quickly but accurately, and use the darned thing on him/her. These devices are pivotally placed for public access should an unfortunate event occur. They're user-friendly. Use it whether you're trained or not! Just be sure to follow the directions. Don't be Dr. Kildare... Or? "Bones" McCoy? Hawkeye Pierce? Doogie Howser? Okay, okay, Dr. McDreamy! FOLLOW THE DIRECTIONS INSIDE THE CASE! According to Jamie Carter, Hampshire County, West Virginia, deputy sheriff, "Most AEDs give voice prompts telling you what to do as soon as you turn it on. They walk you through every step. It won't let you shock someone that doesn't 'need' shocked." Thanks, Jamie!

When you go to the doctor, tell him/her or her/him, anyway, tell everything that is going on with you. Don't play games or hide details or try to guess which part the doctor might want to know. Often the parts you don't tell might help with your diagnosis. And don't be shy around them. Yes, they went to college a long time and deserve that respect; but they, like you, still put their undies on one leg at a time. Do you hear me? You've got THIS book! And unfortunately, cancer sucks, and you don't know when it'll raise its ugly head. Or heart problems. Or something else worthwhile. Unfortunately, many of us are in THAT age group. Sorry.

Also, keep a list of all the products you take or use (including prescription/nonprescription drugs and herbal products) and share it with your doctor and pharmacist. (WebMD) In fact, carry it with you because you never know when it might be needed...and you might be unconscious and unable to give it verbally. Or be like me and forget everything but your name in stressful situations... Okay, you even forget that? Carry your driver's license.

So I went to the most *fabuloso* Doobie Brothers / Santana concert for my 66th birthday. I STILL like it loud like my mother always fussed about way back. SHE SAID I'D GO DEAF... HOWEVER, I might have benefitted from a stern warning from her to not almost fall ass over teacup into the row below us. Heck, in my "other" life, even with no grace—the 3 inch platform shoes that Erma Bombeck said in *Cherries* "brought about dizziness and nosebleeds"—and no handrail, I made it the whole way to the nosebleed section of the West Virginia University Coliseum for a concert in 1974 with no ill effects. What changed?

DIABETES is a very serious and costly disease, which has the potential to affect every part of your body (see "Eyes"). It is a disease with a variety of types that affect how your body uses blood sugar/glucose, an important source of energy for the muscle and tissue cells. Research has shown that those who learn to manage their blood glucose (sugar) levels by eating a healthy diet and exercising regularly can lower their risks of complications and lead a healthier and more productive life. **Insulin** may be prescribed to correct your problem. It is important to take this seriously because failure to do so may lead to damage to the toes, feet, and legs, which may need to be removed a little at a time. Internal organs can be seriously damaged also. With our increasingly poor diets due to fast and junk foods, obesity is on the rise also. It is directly connected to higher incidences of diabetes. If you're running to the bathroom more frequently, that's a red flag for diabetes. Be checked. But...panic not! Health departments, hospitals, and county extension services, to name a few, provide seminars and workshops on how to cope with it. Some even offer COOKING LESSONS. My personal favorite, *Dining with Diabetes*, "offers information, recipes, and tastings" (*Cumberland Times-News*).

Also...okay, it's a BIG aging issue! This is from Jill Weisenberger, registered dietician and author of *Prediabetes: A Complete Guide*:

> Since it's tougher to absorb certain nutrients as we age, make sure to include **protein** to prevent muscle loss, **lutein** for your eyesight and **magnesium** for healthy blood pressure. [Writer's note—When taken just prior to bedtime, magnesium can help to prevent nighttime leg cramps.]

Additionally, the **National Institutes of Health and Academy of Nutrition and Dietetics** recommend that your diet have

Calcium—1,000-1,200 milligrams per day

Potassium—2,600-3,400 milligrams per day
Fiber—25-38 grams per day
Vitamin B12—2.4 micrograms per day
Vitamin D—600 IU per day

These can be purchased over-the-counter to supplement your diet, if you're just not sure you're making the grade. (Sheryl Kraft, "How to Manage Your Weight after 50," *Parade*, Sunday, February 9, 2020)

My brain cells, skin cells, and hair cells continue to die. But my stubborn fat cells seem to have eternal life. (Facebook)

I'm getting real sick and tired of food having calories. (Facebook)

It's all games until your metabolism slows down. (Facebook)

IF you only eat at buffet bars, you will get fat. End of subject. Well, wait, IF you eat more than you should and are sedentary, you will get fat, buffets or not. There's more. IF you continue to eat at your high-school, football-playing pace as you age, you WILL get fat. IF you do not acknowledge (with amazement) the amount you used to eat when your metabolism worked harder, you're probably gonna get FAT! And like it or not, fatness is associated with lots of health problems.

Blue Zones around the world are homes to the highest percentages of centenarians. Healthy diets full of beans, legumes, nuts, whole grains, spinach, and avocadoes seem to play an important part in helping these people live longer, healthier lives. This lifestyle also includes regular exercise, moderate amounts of alcohol, enough sleep, and good spiritual, family, and social participation. Dan Buettner's new cookbook, *The Blue Zones Kitchen*, contains tasty, nutritious recipes from these zones. ("What America Eats," *Parade*, January 12, 2020)

According to *The Kane Show* on iHeartRADIO, "Drinking beer daily can almost double a man's chances of hitting 90. And it increases women's chances by about one-third." I love radio!

Don't eat certain foods at night, or you'll find them helping you count your sheep! Heck, don't eat close to bedtime. Ideally you shouldn't eat after 6:00 p.m.!

Another article from *Parade* slaps the silly out of those who haven't already realized:

> Because dietary needs and the ability to utilize and absorb nutrients change with age, it's more important than ever to focus on a high-quality diet once you reach your **50s**.

And they offer 4 expert-approved diets which, along with 30 minutes of aerobic exercise and strength training, should help to manage your weight after 50. They are the following:

Intermittent fasting—This is not eating for a certain number of hours during the 24-hour day. Their suggestion appealed to me. They suggested not eating between 8:00 p.m. and noon. Being asleep easing some of the temptation time is the way I thought of it! During this time, the body goes into its fat stores for energy. BINGO! Along with reducing several health risks, it can help to prevent diabetes, and the one that jumped out at me was that it can protect memory! HOLY MACKEREL! But that's 16 hours from a 24-hour day with no FOOD! No wonder you'd lose weight!

DASH Diet—The main goal is to reduce blood pressure by cutting sodium in the diet. Recommended eating habits include whole grains, low-fat dairy, fruits and vegetables, and some fish, poultry, legumes, nuts, and seeds. My concern with this one is that it would be easy to not get enough protein.

WW—Guess what, it's Weight Watchers in disguise! Foods are assigned points, and the program for you is customized FOR YOU! No foods are forbidden, nor are any required. The social interaction / support of this program seems to help with long-term success. It can stabilize blood sugar and lower blood pressure.

Mediterranean diet—This is just a very sensible plant-based diet using fruits, vegetables, whole grains, beans, nuts, and seeds, with fish, seafood, and healthy fats, like olive oil, AND dairy, eggs, poultry, AND RED WINE (2 glasses per day for men and 1 per day for women)! Eat reasonably sized portions. This one has been proven to increase life span and promote healthy aging.

Pick one!

After all of that, there is nothing at all wrong with being a larger more curvaceous woman. It's just nature's way of saying, "OMG, you're so bloody good I made more of You!" (Facebook)

I am not heavy. I am a Substantial Woman!

It seems that, upon waking, one does a quick assessment of which parts hurt and prioritizes said pain, then do a few stretches to find as yet undiscovered surprises and to possibly eliminate them before getting up. OMIGOODNESS! My finger was bent at a 90-degree angle rather than its normal 180! It didn't hurt, but what the heck happened while I snoozed? It was **trigger finger**, I soon learned. And the darned thing continued for months until it was actually quite painful. Funny-looking thing.

Solution? Give it an injection. No problem, I thought. However, that sucker hurt like a son of a gun when the doctor used what felt like a half-inch diameter drill bit!

Result—The finger returned to painless, normal function. For how long? Remember that baa-doop, baa-doop lurking tone from *Jaws*?

Don't worry too much if your hands develop a tremor. However, it's a good idea to mention this to your physician at your annual checkup, just in case you have other symptoms also that could indicate **multiple sclerosis** or **Parkinson's disease**.

Multiple sclerosis, commonly referred to as MS, is indicated by the following:

1. Numbness and tingling
2. Muscle spasms
3. Vertigo and dizziness
4. Bladder and bowel problems
5. Abnormal vision
6. Fatigue
7. Memory loss
8. Sexual problems
9. Depression
10. Seizures

Parkinson's Disease—Unfortunately, this is another malady that may show up during the aging process. The **Parkinson's Foundation** offers these 10 early signs of the disease:

1. Tremor
2. Smaller-than-usual handwriting
3. Loss of smell
4. Trouble sleeping
5. Trouble moving or walking
6. Constipation
7. A softer or lower voice
8. Masked face
9. Dizziness or fainting
10. Stooping or hunching over

Individually these signs could apply to lots of other conditions, but when a cluster of them gathers in a person, it would be timely to check with your general practitioner, who will likely send you to a neurologist to set up your plan of action for managing it.

Available through the Michael J. Fox Foundation for Parkinson's Research is this cognitive changes guide by Rachel Dolhoun, MD, *Navigating Cognitive Changes in Parkinson's Disease*. Michael J. Fox is a well-known actor (sitcom: *Family Ties*; movie: *Back to the Future*; TV: *The Good Wife*) who was diagnosed with Parkinson's in 1991 at age 29 and continues to work despite progression of the disease.

My tremor just showed up one day, probably due to stress overload. I came to find out from my neurologist, finally, that it's called an essential tremor and that it's probably genetic. It's a pain for needle threading, TYPING, putting on straight lipstick, and things like that; so I don't see why it's so essential!

Around <u>my</u> age of 30, Mother used to pummel me with remarks about dressing age appropriately. With alarm, in my mind's eye, I saw myself DOOMED to a life of matronly attire. Having been a Chubettes child / large teen in a small-clothes world, I abhorred matronly clothes! THEREFORE, I will go to my GRAVE, despite—or because of—my mother's warning, wearing EXACTLY what I please, be it short or long or BRIGHT! Although I think I may be doing damage to the public when I wear short skirts. Heck, short ANYTHING!

Oh, yes, but clothing has to feel comfortable and breathe. As my former mother-in-law, Dawn, rest her soul, cautioned me in the 70s, polyester doesn't breathe and is hot; cotton and natural fabrics do and are cooler. And that's never changed in 40-something years. Be aware that many garments, especially for "older" or plus-sized women, are made of polyester; so it can stretch. Now, if I'm having a hot splash, the LAST thing I want on me is something that doesn't breathe; fat HAS to breathe! Did I just say that? Go ahead; laugh at me. O, and it smears your glasses worse when you try to clean them with it!

> When you don't dress like everybody else, you don't have to think like everybody else. (Iris Apfel, fashion icon well into her nineties)

> Young'uns-Beware of HOT FLASHES/POWER SURGES/ OR I-WANNA-MELT moments. They just may be God's way of warning us about hell! (Facebook)

Regarding HOT SPLASHES, they are usually—but not always—part of MENOPAUSE, which typically occurs in the late forties but can be anytime when periods slow down or stop, along with a ton of other changes I'll leave to your gynecologist. But WebMD gives these menopause symptoms:

— Uneven or missed periods—Always fun. You never know when there's gonna be a pop-up to ruin your day…or clothes.
— Vaginal dryness—Visit WM for some lubricant. They make men's and women's tingly stuff. Don't ask.
— Sore breasts—Can be VERY uncomfortable!
— Needing to pee more often—Great…
— Trouble sleeping—NOOOOO, especially when you're working!
— Emotional changes—Time for husbands and other significants to take shelter.
— Dry skin, eyes, or mouth—EVERYTHING dries up! Are there no benefits?

Well, once you survive this, you won't have to worry about pregnancy ANYMORE! Birth control no more! Unless you're one of those ones who THINKS it's over...but it's not quite... and in your 40s—or, God forbid, 50s—you're doing diapers again when you've been planning your retirement. God, this part of a woman's life, starting with periods, is just not fun or funny.

Hot splashes do not always end when menopause does. In fact, those rascals can end and start again at any time. Of course, all the doctors excuse them to hormones. I am here to tell you that's not the only cause! Stress, medications, pain, and other mysterious factors could be to blame. Check it out first with your GYN to determine or rule out hormones so you can tell the doctors to dig harder. Do not be ignored. Advocate for yourself always when it comes to medical issues. Oh, and have your annual or, as recommended, mammograms, PAP smears, and pelvic exams!

When women get a certain age, they start accumulating dogs. This is known as "many paws." (Facebook)

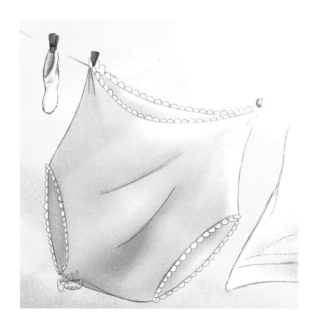

Ever heard of a "dunlop"? It's when your belly's dun lopped over. It wasn't there before. And nobody tells you it's gonna happen! But there it is, precipitating the move from high cuts to briefs (otherwise known as GRANNY PANTIES, echoes of Bridget Jones) to cover the mess! My late sister, whom I assume had similar genes, elected to continue wearing her bikinis. NOW, I know the absolute need for GRANNY PANTIES! AND GUYS! Omigoodness, have you noticed how far DOWN their dunlops can shove their pants in the front? Well, they can be practically down to the point of NO return! I don't want THAT spilling out in a nice restaurant! I tell Kenny his belt is vertical and to watch it! But it is funny to imagine the belt size of some of those big dudes! The belt under the bulge (the belly!) is like a 32! If the girth was rounded by a tape measure, it would read more like 46!

Birthdays have a way of creeping up on you. They're kinda like granny panties that way.

As one's size changes and/or parts shift, and they inevitably will, get rid of clothes you've been storing away. You aren't likely to magically be able to wear those things again. Or by the time you're able to, they'll be way out of style! Or you'll be in nightgowns in a home somewhere! Donate them to your local thrift store, but make sure the one you use has an honest history of giving back to the community.

Vignette

Helping Hands is our local thrift store *exceptionale*. Most items sell for $0.10 to $1.00. It's easy to carry out a whole bagful of goodies having spent less than $5.00! Women go in to treasure hunt. Men go shopping for "new" clothes for some event, like a funeral, theirs or others. Kids raid the joint for new toys, clothes, and school project materials, and it's a great source of holiday whatnots.

Because it was within walking distance, Ian and Kathy visited weekly—or more often if they got bored, I'm convinced. However, one of the most hallowed uses of HH clothing was the time, years ago, when a certain few bored, well-known youth dressed the WWI doughboy statue in front of the courthouse in LOVELY lingerie in the middle of the night when their parents thought they were safely in bed. A close 2nd occurred when the large evergreen tree next to the doughboy was decorated with a color variety of bras for October's Breast Cancer Awareness Month!

Oh, and FYI, income for the year at Helping Hands is usually between $50,000 and $70,000, which is gifted to multiple service organizations in the area, like the volunteer fire companies. HH does this EVERY year with volunteer service and volunteer item donations.

> When you retire, don't just sit down 'cause you're gonna die. Use your experience and time you have left to make a difference. VOLUNTEER! You'll meet new people and have new experiences. This is my theory on avoiding Alzheimer's. (Ms. Helping Hands, Diana, age 72)

One more nag about smoking, it doesn't matter when you stop; there already is damage to your lungs for the time that you did. (This came from a real doctor.) And COPD resulting from this, and some other things, limits a person. Who wants to carry around an oxygen pocketbook wherever they go and worry whether it'll run out before they get home? And yes, it's big enough to be a pocketbook, not a purse.

> Fact—About 30 percent of Americans who have had **chicken pox** develop **SHINGLES**, with the risk increasing with increasing age. (Patrick Turnes, MD, *Hampshire Review*, Romney, West Virginia, September 25, 2019, page 7C)

> Shingles causes a painful rash that may appear as a strip of blisters usually on the face or trunk of the body. Pain can persist even after the rash is gone. (Mayo Clinic)

A preventative vaccine is available and should be seriously considered.

I remember my elderly great, great-aunt suffering miserably with a track of shingles that went down her forehead and onto her eyelid! I also remember my plucky mother-in-law self-medicating before she knew what she had—with Icy Hot. The spot ached; she took care of it. As we laughed about it, in the back of our minds, we were wondering if IH maybe did help. She seemed to pass through it pretty well.

However, Gretchen (Lizzy, I've called her since childhood), age 40, has had a MISER-ABLE time:

I was told that shingles was a condition that people in their fifties and sixties were at risk of getting. In fact, shingles vaccines aren't even approved unless you are fifty years old or older. Unfortunately I turned forty this year, and I have had to experience this condition in its fiercest form! Five days after I had a surgical procedure, I began to have weakness in my arms and legs along with full-body twitching. I had test after test, which ruled out multiple sclerosis (MS), amyotrophic lateral sclerosis (ALS), and/or other neurological conditions but gave me no answer to what I had. After about six weeks, these symptoms faded. I was ecstatic about starting to feel better. Five days later, I began developing a severe earache. The urgent-care center diagnosed inner and outer ear infections. I googled it, of course, and found that it can be "waited out" to avoid taking antibiotics. So I did that. On the fifth day, it became unbearable, and my hearing became muffled. And I developed a fever, aches, and chills. The doctor put me on antibiotics. The following day, as I was running an errand, water dribbled down my chin when I took a drink; and I had the sensation of receiving Novocain at the dentist. A horrifying look in my rearview mirror confirmed that my face was drooping on the affected ear side as though I'd had a stroke. At the ER, it was determined that I had not had a stroke or an ear infection. I had shingles on my 7th cranial nerve, known as Ramsay Hunt syndrome. This does not always present with blisters, and obviously being forty didn't mean anything to it either. Even with a dose of antivirals, over the next several days, the pain increased. The paralysis became worse, and my hearing faded almost completely in the affected ear. It was confirmed by an ENT that I had significant neurological hearing loss. This yielded a high dose of steroids in the hope of relieving the inflammation and pressure on my cranial nerve. I was informed that, without them, I was at risk of having **permanent** damage. Over the next six weeks, with bedrest for extreme pain and feeling very ill, my hearing greatly improved; and the paralysis improved by 80 percent. Unfortunately, each time I finished a dose of antivirals, the shingles infection reared its ugly head again.

I continue to have significant ear pain. Ramsay Hunt can sadly last for years with lingering facial nerve and ear pain, paralysis, and hearing loss. A compassionate doctor familiar with the condition is definitely needed for the ongoing care. RH is said to affect 5 out of every 100,000 people. I am thinking, with my luck, I should play the lottery!

Prostatectomy—HAHAHA. Funny word. Uh-oh, not funny. Not funny at all! Men, get that rascal prostate checked just as often as your doctor tells you! The exam is only really not funny for a minute or two, but the BIG WORD means SURGERY.

Nearly all men die WITH prostate cancer, but few die FROM prostate cancer. (From a family physician a while back)

Men, according to several TV channels, if your banana starts looking like a banana pepper, or your banana pepper starts looking like a carrot, or your carrot starts looking like—well, you get the picture—get it checked. It could have Peyronie's disease, which comes from scar tissue. Don't ask me! I'm just the relayer! I know, ladies. Now, all your men will be checking down there looking for crooks and turns.

Strong men are smart men when they know asking for help doesn't minimize anything.

When you reach the stage that you cannot do some things or you shouldn't be doing certain things, like climbing ladders or moving wood, get some help! There will always, hopefully, be kids who need a little spending money or are saving for college. Sensibly share the wealth and save yourself. (O! I made a rhyme!)

If I had thought I'd live this long, I'd have taken better care of my parts!

Parts should be given warrantees like cars. I mean, when the wheels stop wheelin' and the radiator quits radiating and the pistons—well, you know—stop doin' whatever they do, you need to get them repaired or replaced.

Beware: age yields **arthritis**, **bunions**, **hammertoes**, crossed toes, knobby fingers, diminished eyesight and hearing, and on and on. Be prepared to resize your rings, get wider shoes, invest in good hearing aids, sit down to hold kids and pets, and have cataract surgery. HOWEVER, you WILL still be able to hold your grandchildren and great-grands.

Become friends with **BENGAY**, **Poligrip**, **Gold Bond Extreme Healing and crepiness**, **Bag Balm** (of course, it's real), EVERY bathroom EVER constructed and where it's located, pencil grips, built-up silverware, jar openers with handles, l-o-n-g shoehorns, grabbers for picking up stuff you have trouble reaching (Kenny used his to remove a little snake from our house after his hip surgery), sock pullers, buttoning tools, magnetic necklace clasps, and zipper pulls. Okay, maybe I got carried away, but the goal is being able to do it yourself and not needing help as you're really aging. These become especially important if you live alone.

Rule of Thumb: Always "go" when you see one because "holding it" is no longer an option! Commit to memory that the following words mean "bathroom": ladies, loo, cowgirls, *die toilette* (German), *el cuarto* (Spanish), *toilette* (Italian), and *toilette* (French). And when traveling outside this country, you may find them in fast-food restaurants, hotel lobbies, department stores, in buildings in the middle of the sidewalk, or railway and bus stations.

When I was little, I laughed when my aunt crossed her legs when she coughed. I no longer find that funny.

However, rest assured that, just as menstrual pads occur, so do bladder control products for women (and men) and in the same section much of the time. So as the ads on TV say, something like this, "Oh, I used to be so worried that my control product might be obvious, but now I'm FREE because they're so improved that they won't show!" I'd still be a tad cautious wearing those "beautiful briefs" under thin polyester pants that are too tight or leggings...in beige, which is another whole discussion topic in itself. **OH**, but according to the **Because** ad, "New protective underwear allows seniors to live free again." Paints a couple of pictures, doesn't it?

Now I've been going to the restroom by myself for quite a long time. Open the door, go in, do my thing, out the door, and WASH MY HANDS (A personal observation is that not all feel this step is necessary—YUCK! One of these days, or several, I'm going to park myself at the sink / bathroom door in a variety of public restrooms and do a count on who does and who doesn't! Then I'm gonna publish it somewhere, like a public health magazine or, better yet, in a restaurant guide of some sort. Heck, I could just do it for the Golden M and paste it on the windows! Or the WM place and ask for a special on hand sanitizer.

Okay, okay, I'm too passionate about it). But hey, those wider-door public restroom stalls with grab rails are pretty tempting...just in case I'd take a dipsy-doodle, as my mother called her falls. HECK, there's room in there for the EMTs and gurneys and spectators!

Advice: most people, as they age, do not naturally get unusually loopier in a short time, like I am; so if they are, or you are, get a **urinalysis**! Urine/bladder infections can occur more frequently with aging. And there have been some pretty wacky people in nursing homes written off as losing it, and given drugs, before a urinary infection was discovered.

WAIT...it's white DOWN THERE, too?
What? Is that thing shrinking?
Do people have sex after midlife? Let's ask those who are having a lively good time with new partners...after YEARS of NOTHING. OF COURSE, THEY DO! Even your parents did (at least until your mother said that was enough of that stuff after 50 or so years), BUT...evidently men's sexual urges NEVER go away. Guess they have to regularly drain the smaller of the 2 heads so their brains can function in the larger of the two. Oops, TMI?
Think lubricant—LOTS of lubricant! Seriously, because "things" lose their natural moisture during menopause. YIPPEE! One more menopause associated s-l-i-d-e.

Parts you can afford to lose if necessary:

1. Tonsils
2. Appendix
3. Gall bladder
4. Toenails
5. Fingernails
6. Uterus
7. Ovaries
8. One kidney
9. Part of your stomach or liver
10. Hair

After that, take under due consideration any other removals your doctor might mention.

Yucky but factual—IF **YOUR POOP'S BLACK**, go to the ER IMMEDIATELY! This indicates blood loss somewhere in those great entrails of yours!

At a formal dinner party, the person nearest death should always be seated closest to the bathroom. (George Carlin, American comedian)

Theory:

I understand why we fall apart as we age. Because I believe it's God's way so that, when it's time to leave, we're ready to go. Because, if we felt as good as we did when we were 18, we would never want to go…and we'd fight it. (Dr. Heather, age 67, GEN I US!)

It's scary to think that, one day, we're going to have to live without our mother or father, or brother, or husband or wife or that, one day, we're going to have to walk this earth without our best friend by our side or them without us. Appreciate your loved ones while you can because none of us is going to be here forever. (Facebook)

A dying parent means realizing that the earthly body you've loved fiercely will soon be one with the earth. If we were fortunate growing up, we all relied heavily on our parents, depending on them to teach us how to get through life, in general. What would we have done without them? As we get older and busier, we tend to stop paying so much attention to them, but we forget they're growing older too, and now's the time that they actually need us to lean on. It's never easy to lose someone you love, and it's especially harder when it's your parents and the only thing that can attenuate is time as it passes. It never really gets better; it's just that you learn to live with the dull pain.

Also, in today's time, it is not possible to stay at home and take care of your ill parent 24/7. No, it's not because you don't love them; it's because you have other commitments, like work.

Shuttling between work, home, and keeping tabs on your parents' conditions can be exhausting, both physically and mentally. Plus, there's that fact that you're always worried about how your parent's health is, wondering if it's improving or deteriorating, and that's painful.

You will hear your dying parent say, "I'm ready," and even though you aren't, you'll let go of the hand that you've held since you were small. When your parent finally finds peace, you realize that your parent is still teaching you about life. (Christine Burke, writer for *Scary Mommy* blog, Facebook)

To care for those who once cared for us is one of life's highest honors. (Facebook)

Keep in mind that, if the frustrations of care or the decline in the person you care for get to be more than you can handle, HOSPICE is wonderful and available for situations like this. Our experience with them was that they were caring medical staff who took much of the hard decision-making out of our hands after consulting with us and took over some of the tough stuff, like bathing, turning the person, and catheter and colostomy care. Senior services also offer valuable assistance and usually transport options for seniors. As Dad's dementia progressed, he attended a day program that was a godsend for my mother as she attempted to keep him home as long as possible.

In the Sioux tribe tradition, older members are honored and taken care of by all. "Our teachings are in place but not in as many homes as we'd like. Our elders are regarded as the wisdom keepers and the keys to all the mysterious doorways that have been left for us by our ancestors. Our elders are considered to be the closest to the Creator like a baby when it was first given to us as a gift to be on Mother Earth." (Galena Rose Drapeau, *Dakota Way of Life Keeper*)

As I get older and remember all the people I've lost along the way, I think perhaps I wasn't the best tour guide. (Pastor Roy, age 67)

I saw an ad for a coffin and thought, "That's the last thing I need." (Pastor Roy, age 67)

Vignette

Pastor Roy is the minister for my age group because he's one of us. I don't mean he's old; but he carries many of the same values, views, and memories we've saved from the '60s and '70s. They are just imbedded in us. Oh, and he's a little nuts—like the rest of us. I like that.

When someone dies, there are BURIAL OPTIONS, as offered by Carter Wagoner, Shaffer Funeral Home, Romney, West Virginia:

Every time you get dressed, remember that, if you die, that's going to be your ghost outfit forever. (Comments on Carter's news feed, Facebook)

— Cremation—The body is reduced to ashes, which you may have for remembrance, to deposit where you choose, or to be included in jewelry in wee bits, or to be pressurized into diamonds (?) or other interesting choices.

Heck, if you die and get cremated, you can be put in an hourglass and still be in on family game night. (Comments on Carter's news feed, Facebook; just make sure they strain out the chunks or you could still be accused of cheating!)

Regarding cremation, that's my last hope for a smokin' hot body! (Comments on Carter's news feed, Facebook)

— Burial without embalming—This is another option, but it must be done within 2–3 days of death. Many times, in years past, the deceased was cleaned up, dressed, and put on display on the dining room table or in the parlor. One of Kenny's FAVORITE Ray Stevens songs/videos is "Sitting Up with the Dead." The lyrics of which are worth looking up! Just a hint, he says, "I stopped sitting up with the dead when the dead started sitting up too." Ray Stevens is an American singer/songwriter/comedian. (Sorry. I got distracted.)

— Burial with embalming—The bodily fluids are removed and replaced with preserving fluid, thereby allowing a longer period of time for visitation and burial.

— Burial without embalming—We found that this can be a choice when my sister died. As long as guidelines for being within a few days are followed, it may be done.

No casket, no cost; Tennesseans go back to "natural" burial. [What the heck?] It's a "green" cemetery, which its operators say means people buried there can't be embalmed or placed in a casket. People can dig their own grave, place a loved one in it, and cover it themselves. (Justin McDuffie, Maggie Gregg, and Nick Viviani, WVLT / Gray News, February 20, 2020)

As of April 2020, this is being offered using a biodegradable "box" by our Romney mortuary, Shaffer Funeral Home, with burial in a special section of our local cemetery. (*Hampshire Review Weekender*, April 2020)

You may bury on your own property as long as you are not within 100 feet of a water source. (Carter Wagoner, owner / funeral director, age 62)

You know you're getting old when you realize that 75 years ago, doctors who looked at people your age were called coroners. (*Old Jokes for Old Folks*)

When I die, I want to die like my grandfather who died peacefully in his sleep, not screaming like all the passengers in his car. (Will Rogers, American film actor)

Love the people God sent you; one day, He'll need them back.

Whereas ye know not what *shall* be on the morrow. For what *is* your life? It is even a vapour, that appeareth for a little time, and then vanisheth away. (James 4:14 KJV)

Dust in the wind
All we are is dust in the wind
(Kansas, rock band, "Dust in the Wind")

Be humble and never think that you are better than anyone else, and unto dust you shall return. (Facebook)

This reminded me of my dad and my first trip to the cemetery after his burial. There it was—a mound of dirt. He left, and all there was to show for his physical life was a pile of dirt. All that harping about money and nastiness and hard times he gave us still led to nothing but a heap of dirt, just like everybody else. So why did we have to go through life with him as we did?

Ashes to ashes, dust to dust
It'll never be the same
But we're all forgiven
We're only living
To leave the way we came.
(The Fifth Dimension, American music group)

A dear friend of ours died from COVID in February 2021. It was an intensely desperate time, and I said to another friend of hers, "How will we live without Janet?" (Because she was such a valuable person in so many parts of our lives, especially our summer school mission project to the Lakota Sioux Reservation in South Dakota.) Our extremely wise and gifted Sylvia said to me, "She will live on through us in the ways she affected us. She'll never be gone." (Janet called us her "pod.")

As I've studied that comment, I realize this is similar to the story of the stone (our actions) thrown in the water that creates ripples that continue on and on.

And Roy, whom I've mentioned earlier, presented in a funeral yesterday that a mother (anyone) is like a tree that drops its apples in the fall, which become trees in the spring; and the cycle goes on and on.

We all affect those with whom we come in contact, and we pass much of life on to future generations.

> One day, you'll be just a memory for some people. Do your best to be a good one. (Facebook)

Be sure to focus on what will REALLY make a difference when you're gone.

> Your life is a movie, playing out second by second, frame by frame. So how will you fill that time? And will it be worth replaying in your mind over and over again? (Inspirato, luxury vacation homes, TV Commercial, 2020)

> Pass on valuable skills to those who follow. (Reverend Mark, age 57)

> Love your life. Take pictures of everything. Tell people you love them. Talk to random strangers. Do things that you're scared to do. So many of us die, and no one remembers a thing we did. Take your life and make it the best story in the world. Don't waste it. (Facebook)

I've told Ian that, when I die, I'd like for them to have a party and tell goofy stories about my life. Hmmm, they better plan a lot of food...and maybe hotel reservations. Heck knows there's been a lot of stuff!

> Time is like a river. You cannot touch the same water twice, because the flow that has passed will never pass again. Enjoy every moment in life! (John Tesh, American performer and TV personality)

> Therefore we do not lose heart. Though outwardly we are wasting away, yet inwardly we are being renewed day by day. (2 Corinthians 4:16 NIV)

According to an article by Eleanor Cummins in **Vox** on January 22, 2020, Millennials are the "death-positive" generation. Younger people are planning their own funerals. And that's creating change in the death business. As healthy 20 somethings, they're signing papers to donate their bodies to science FAAAR down the road. Apparently, after the research is finished, universities will cremate the bodies when they're finished their studies and return the ashes to the family, thereby preventing a financial burden to the family.

Continuing the Cummins article, research in 2017 found that only 1 in 3 adults in the US has end-of-live directives. Only 21 percent of Americans have even discussed their passing with their families, according to the National Funeral Directors Association. GET ON IT! There is unlimited internet information on the subject right down to having your ashes turned into diamonds (YouTube "Ask a Mortician") if you so desire. Check this article for more good information. WHAT ARE YOU WAITING FOR? OKAY! For what are you waiting? Just do it!

Do your **living will** (Don't know what this is? Find out!) LONG before you think you'll need it and post it on the fridge where EMTs look when they come in. That's what they told me when I needed Mother's. It was locked up in the safe deposit box on a SUNDAY (Mother was like that with important stuff), and I had no options but to remove the intubation tube down her throat myself. She precisely did not want that kind of thing. Don't leave your family (sibs are known to have huge fights over what to do) hanging on these life-and-death situations.

Also, make your ORGAN DONOR decisions yourself. Have this indicated on your driver's license, if available. Make your family aware and put it in your living will. According to Facebook on April 30, 2020, more than 450 relatives of organ donors declined permission to donate as they were unsure of their relatives' wishes in 2018. Granted Facebook may be an unreliable source, but don't put your family in the position to have to make this decision.

> As soon as you die, your identity becomes a "**body**." People use the phrases like "Bring the **body**," "Lower the **body** in the grave," "Take the **body** to the graveyard," etc. People don't even call you by your name whom you tried to impress [your] whole life. Live a life to impress the Creator, not the creation. (Facebook)

I can't quote the book
You can't tell me it all ends
In a slow ride in a hearse
You know I'm more and more convinced
The longer that I live
Yeah, this can't be, no, this can't be
No, this can't be all there is
Lord, I raise my hands
Bow my head
Oh, I'm findin' more and more truth
In the words written in red
They tell me that there's more to life
Than just what I can see, I believe.
(Brooks and Dunn, musical duo, "Believe")

Jeanne Louise Calment, a French lady, had the oldest documented life span of 122 years and 164 days. She died in 1997. Here are her Rules of Life:
"I'm in love with wine."
"All babies are beautiful."
"I think I will die of laughter."
"I've been forgotten by our Good Lord."
"I've got only one wrinkle, and I'm sitting on it."
"I never wear mascara; I laugh until I cry often."
"If you can't change something, don't worry about it."
"Always keep your smile. That's how I explain my long life."
"I see badly, I hear badly, and I feel bad, but everything's fine."
"I have a huge desire to live and a big appetite, especially sweets (including chocolate)."
"I have legs of iron, but to tell you the truth, they're starting to rust and buckle a bit."
"I took pleasure when I could. I acted clearly and morally and without regret. I'm very lucky."
"Being young is a state of mind, it doesn't depend on one's body. I'm actually still a young girl, it's just that I haven't looked so good for the past 70 years."
Amen.

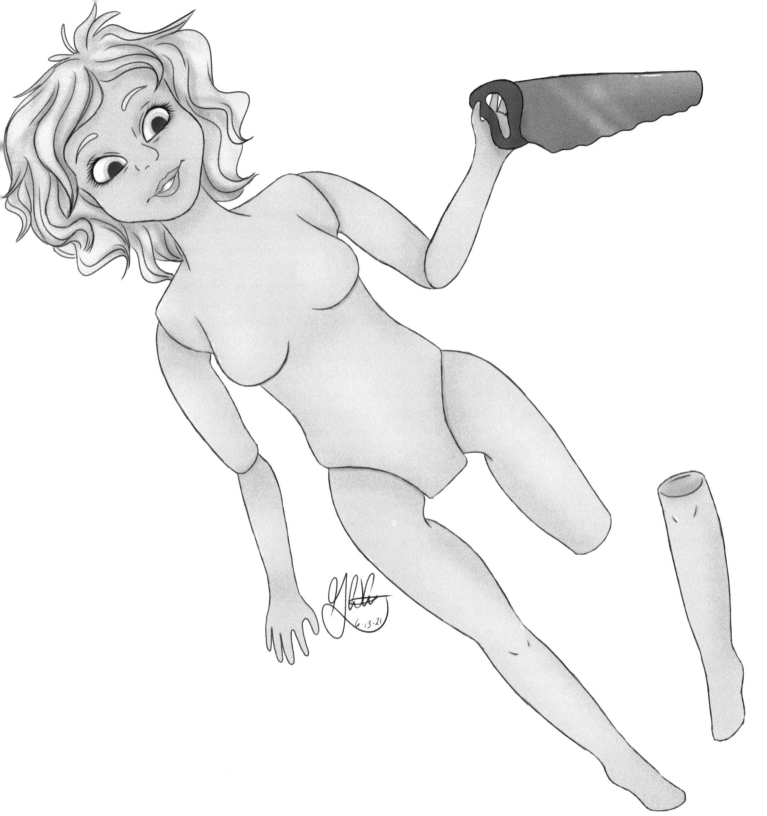

Mobility

The inevitable—you will inevitably end up groaning or grunting when you stand up...like the rest of us. Get used to it.

> I asked Kay one day if she remembered what it was like to move without sound effects. (Thelma, age 70)

> Keep moving. (Howard, age 63)

> I'm inspired by people who keep on rolling, no matter their age. (Jimmy Buffett, musician)

In a rapid-fire stream that he says comes from being a New Englander, when asked about aging, my doctor spit out that he no longer runs like the wind on the jetties. Nor does he vault from a pickup bed without realizing something is different. He's not sure whether it's that he's not as dumb as he used to be or if his body is trying to communicate something else to him. He also got mortally offended when his wife told him that the girl at the gym who asked him to spot her, rather than asking the "big" guys, probably felt he was "a safe older man," or something like that. You get the sentiment. He was amused but not particularly thrilled. (Dr. Ed, age 56)

Collection of thoughts from the sage Kay P., age 75:

In the general course of things, we tend to be very self-absorbed; but as we get older and our lives are disordered by our various trials, we realize just how important it is to support one another. We are of an age that some consider old; I prefer to think we're experienced. We appreciate each other so much that we do sometimes get a little pushy with our caring (which she let me know in a confusing but firm manner in winter 2021!). Our purpose is to care for one another.

Also, think ahead; plan ahead. Impulse is a gift given to youth. It can turn deadly with an aging body. If you are going to the grocery store, you go from one aisle to the next and review your list (writer's note—MAKE LISTS...for lots of things, and don't lose them; they'll cut your frustration as your memory banks become too full and can't hold things as well) as you go.

Plan your daily activities as if you are an UPS driver—line up the things to do, no LEFT turns, don't cross the traffic lanes. Obey the signals your body gives you. If your knees hurt or you feel weak, use a cane, vanity be damned. At best, it can save a disastrous fall. At worst, it's a conversation starter.

Finally

1. THINK!
2. Common sense in all things (writer's note—hopefully you're born with some).
3. If I had thought I'd live this long, I'd have taken better care of parts!

Vignette

I had no big sister. I was the firstborn. However, over time, I have been adopted by this bossy woman who tells me like it is whether I want to hear it or not! I resent that and would not accept it from anyone else. But she's pretty smart and knows what she's talking about (most of the time), so I allow her to give me verbal thrashings when I need them (sometimes unnecessarily, I've discovered). And she's often the first person I run to for technical consultation...even on aging.

INDEPENDENCE—As you age, keep in mind these 6 progressive steps to staying independent longer:

1. You are independent.
2. You <u>are</u> independent using a cane.
3. You <u>are</u> independent using a **quad cane** [4-footed cane].
4. You <u>are</u> independent using a walker.
5. You <u>are</u> independent using a **Rollator.**
6. You <u>are</u> independent using a motorized wheelchair.

Each allows you to take care of yourself longer and be independent. (Robin Dohrman Ayers, special disabilities teacher, age 68)

My mother told me to be a lady. And for her, that meant be your own person, be independent. (Ruth Bader Ginsburg, US Supreme Court justice, one of America's greatest legal advocates for gender equality, still practicing at age 67; fortunately I saw the news clip of her saying this because sadly the country lost her on September 19, 2020)

I've taken up a new activity—pole dancing! It's a lot to remember at first. And the daggone pole is slippery from the soap sometimes. And it's really too big for my hands. But it sure is handy in the shower, and when going uphill, or stepping up into the house.

Be honest. If you're mooring yourself to objects when you're walking—like your closest friend or relative, or walls, or furniture—it might be time to consider getting a cane, walking stick (that's what I'm trying first), or walker. Keep clutter to a minimum (I'm gonna have to move to an empty house!), particularly on stairs, and add grab bars in your shower or bath area and near the toilet. Now it's VERY important to supervise these installations to ensure that you can reach them comfortably. Sit on the toilet and decide where you need them to assist you in getting off the throne. Watch the bath installations. When we redid our bathroom, I went completely into the shower and sat on the bench to determine both height and angle that were best for me. When I got vertigo, I was SO happy that I had them! However, I haven't yet found a use for the one that was installed in my absence, at the wrong side of the door.

And for heaven's sake, OFFER to hold doors for people using crutches, wheelchairs, grocery carts, baby strollers, and such. It is possible to feel disemboweled trying to stretch over those things if you're driving them just to get the daggone door open without hitting what's between you and it! Until one learns that you can go out bum first to push the door, it is quite the challenge! And as for crutches, you almost have to walk in that person's shoes to know the need. Be sure to ASK if someone wants assistance before doing it. Some people will not want the help in their effort to prove that they're still independent / not disabled. That was my sister's thing, and she could be right defensive about it no matter how we tried to calm the beast!

If you have a physical disability or you're finally just not able to walk the half mile to a concert venue (refer to Santana concert) or your feet or knees don't do their job effectively anymore, it is appropriate for you to request a handicapped hangtag or license for your vehicle. See your doctor for the form. You're legit. BUT my rule of thumb is to NOT park in the BIG H if I'm able to walk that day. Somebody else might need it more than I do. But put the renewal date for your state handicap hangtag or license on your "must-remember calendar."

Balance—Be prepared for a thrill ride as you never know what it's gonna be or when it's gonna change or how it's gonna change or where it's gonna challenge you or who's gonna be affected. Sometimes I feel like Arte Johnson (1929-2019) on *Rowan and Martin's Laugh-In*—I'm standing, and suddenly my tricycle's over on its side. And I'm like, with a dumb look on my face, "Velllly intelesting, but schtupid."

Be aware that VERTIGO is different from regular dizziness! I had VERTIGO, and I swear it was like having a Gremlin inside me! I didn't just fall over (think little old lady, hand to mouth, going "Oops"). NO, this was like a bloody gorilla picking me up and throwing me against walls, floors, and steps and precipitating 2 fun, fun ER trips! (Dr. Heather has had it also and said it was like 2 giant hands on her chest SHOVING her backward.

Thank God, her bed was there.) The cause may be an inner ear thingy or a head bump or God knows what, but be sure to explore ALL options to get rid of it so you don't get hurt! Physical therapy, Dramamine (or prescription meclizine), and physician-prescribed exercises (but NOT the ones MY doctor told me about for ridding myself of it quickly; he said to log roll over and over until I stopped being sick from it… I opted to NOT!) were all run past my head—well, actually, inner ear. PT fixed one ear; BUT I, like not too many other people, had it in BOTH ears. And that second one would NOT clear up. It was so bad that it threw me on a set of steps, bruising a part of my anatomy SO bad that we had to postpone a trip to Mexico! When we finally ventured down south the next month, it (the vertigo) cleared up ON THE PLANE. Perhaps the altitude did it?

> We may be getting older, but that does not mean we have to be boring and act our age. (Facebook)

Dance before the music is over. Live before your life is over. Dancing can reverse the signs of aging in the brain.

> Studies are now showing that dance may just be the number-one activity for protecting and strengthening your brain. There's constant learning. It trains and improves coordination and balance. Memory improves because you're connecting the mental with the physical. Music stimulates brain activity. Dancing makes you happy—exercise, connect with people, and less stressed. (Facebook)

> Just dance to the beat of your soul. (Facebook)

> When you stumble, make it part of the dance. Smile at the crowd, kick up your heels and dance a jig! The moment you embrace it as your own, no one will know it's not part of YOUR dance. (Suzy Toronto, *Life Is All About How You Handle Plan B*)

> Dance even if you are too bad at it. Pose stupidly for photos. Be childlike.

Moral: Death is not the greatest loss in life. Loss is when life dies inside you while you are alive. Celebrate this event called life. (Facebook)

I'M NOT CLUMSY! It's just the floor hates me, the tables and chairs are bullies and the wall gets IN MY WAY! (Facebook)
And they're more than likely gonna get meaner with age—theirs and yours!

Question: Why do lots of older people walk funny? It's kind of a wide-footed waddle going slowly left and right. Could it be any of the following associated with aging?

1. Arthritis
2. Joints—worn-out knees and hips
3. Balance issues
4. Tiredness
5. Fear of falling
6. Poor eyesight

Get used to it, babycakes. There's not much preventive stuff you're likely to do for it...other than exercise...to which I'M allergic!

Back to ARTHRITIS, read up on it. Be familiar with it. And batten your hatches because it's bound to catch up with you somewhere, sometime, and some pain...although it just caught up with my 84-year-old adopted family member **recently**!

Arthritis may lead to KNEE or HIP REPLACEMENT; but sometimes those suckers just wear out from years of abuse—skiing, running, walking, sitting, and crossing legs, which my friend Sarah, who is 68, warned me about when we were in our 20s. However, she didn't cross her legs; she walks, runs, etc. and has few, if any, health problems. At Christmas, she snow sledded with her young grandchildren! I—let's face it—am sedentary. I have new knees (shouldn't I be the one with well-preserved knees of my own?), and what a PRIMITIVE process that is. Should you need new ones, it is not for the squeamish! Heck, they saw the bone off above and below the knee to insert the new, artificial one! Gruesome? Ubetcha. HOWEVER, to those contemplating this surgery, if your pain is bad enough, it's definitely worth it. Just make sure you're committed to the ensuing rehab. And the pain is really the worst just the first 3 or so days. Look at it this way: in a year, you'll never really remember it—hopefully—and you'll be running with the big dogs again. Well, maybe not running.

Did you know that, when shoulders are replaced, at least part of the time, the joint is replaced in reversed positions? Kenny's concern was that his palms would face outward!

> I look at these poor people in this parking lot, and I realize how thankful I should be that I can get around like I do! (Kenny, age 76)

> When I am an old lady, I'm going to leave snacks in little bags on the floor all over the house in case I fall down. (Facebook)

Don't be ignorant. Be ready for the day when these needs are going to be there. If you prefer, start a little at a time, like ensuring you have adequate lighting, cutting down on the clutter, and keeping your vision appointments.

People seem to FALL more as they age, which may be due to vertigo, balance problems, loss of strength, vision and hearing issues, weight gain, and many other age-related lovelies. However, people lose bone mass and density as they age (especially women after menopause), which makes this the primary reason why fractures, falls, and accidents are more prevalent among these populations. This loss of bone mass is due to the fact that, with each passing year, our bones lose calcium, vital amino acids, and other minerals required to provide strength and density to our skeletal system. Dietary habits can make or break (no pun intended) the loss of bone mass. Here are a few of the dietary culprits:

1. Soft drinks—Affect acid / calcium balance. Calcium is lost from the bones.
2. Table salt—Too much, which we generally get from our regular diet alone, leeches calcium from the bones.
3. Excessive caffeine—Leeches calcium from bones.
4. Hydrogenated oils (which are found unbeknownst in many foods)—Destroys Vitamin K, which is essential for strong bones.
5. Wheat bran—Contains high levels of phytates, which can interfere with the absorption of calcium, iron, zinc, and magnesium. Example—wheat bran and milk for breakfast. The calcium is blocked.

Do you notice the common factor?

Along with avoiding the above, adding collagen protein to the diet can help rebuild and strengthen bones. (Facebook)

> Even before the coronavirus pandemic caused forced isolation, falling had become the leading cause of injury-related death in people age 65 [writer's note—there's that number again] years and older. About 3 million older adults wind up in an emergency room each year due to a fall… can experience a marked decrease in their quality of life. (Dr. Elizabeth Ko and Dr. Eve Glazier, "Ask the Doctors," *Cumberland Times-News*, Cumberland, Maryland, September 2020)

Additionally they mention these possible contributors: balance problems, weakness in lower extremities, vision issues, lousy-fitting shoes (we all have them—i.e., bedroom slippers), medications that cause dizziness (or, in my case, dizziness from vertigo and neuropathy; I rubbed a heck of a lot of skin off my foot while test-driving some new boots that will be going back, and I never felt a THING! Anyway…), or hazards in the house, like throw rugs (they call them that because they need to be thrown away!) and electric cords (thank you, Mr. Ayers) and slippery tubs. Outside, there are weather-related problems, like ice, cracks, steps, and lighting. AND THEN there are pets, particularly ones on leashes. In our community, a particularly well-liked fellow died when his head hit rocks after he got tangled in his dog's leash while they took a simple walk. It was awful, but we felt he was heaven bound, if anyone was.

If you live alone or are by yourself a good bit, get an EMERGENCY BUTTON! Do not let pride prevent you from obtaining the one item that might save your life in an emergency. Remember the TV commercials of a person lying on the floor, moaning, "Help. I've fallen, and I can't get up"? Well, no matter how lame that may have sounded, if you fall and break your hip, God only knows when you'll be found! Sure, a cell phone can serve that purpose, IF you have that thing with you instead of being on the cabinet at which you just were standing or on your bedside table when you're tangled up in your walker, thrown against the shower door, in a surgical boot with pins sticking out, and tears in both of your rotator cuffs. And your husband's upstairs. Just saying (October 2020). My mother kept her button on faithfully—off before her shower and right back on afterward—along with all her lotions and creams. Oh, and clothes.

HOWEVER, I depended on the button to be an insurance policy when we went to Maine with friends, and she strongly disagreed with having company at night. Early in our trip, her daytime caregiver found her on the floor where she'd been for HOURS! She did not push her button, which she was wearing, because she forgot...she guessed. The disorientation from that fall and consequential time on the floor seemed to us to be the beginnings of her end. **Lesson learned:** Do not depend on emergency buttons when your little inner voice tells you to override her decision. They are good helpers but not the total solution after a certain point in the aging life.

"Still in the work world," **AARP,** aarp.org, January 16, 2020, has clarified **five myths and facts of older workers and age discrimination.**

1. Myth: Older workers aren't as mentally sharp as younger workers.
   Fact: "Crystallized intelligence," a combination of verbal ability and knowledge from their experiences—older executives have more of this than younger counterparts. This comes from a 2015 study by the American Psychological Association.
2. Myth: Older workers are less productive and are not as reliable as younger workers.
   Fact: Researchers on the subject found that older adults, age 65 to 80, excelled over younger adults, age 20–30, on productivity, reliability, motivation, balanced routine, and stable mood when each group was tested on 12 tasks.
3. Myth: Older people aren't as digitally savvy as younger people.
   Fact: Through recent surveys, the Pew Research Center has found that in the 65-plus age group, two-thirds use the internet, with 75 percent using it daily, 37 percent using social media, and 42 percent using a smartphone.
4. Myth: Dementia is an increasing risk among older Americans.
   Fact: Results of a 12-year study of more than 21,000 people, published in JAMA INTERNAL MEDICINE in 2016, found a decline of 2.8 percent between 2000 and 2012.
5. Myth: Older workers are more ornery (imagine that...) and difficult to get along with.
   Fact: Ashton Applewhite, author of *This Chair Rocks*, believes that Americans 65-plus showed themselves, in a survey by General Social Survey, to be in the

highest percentage of very happy workers due to "greater emotional maturity, adaptability to change, and levels of well-being."

And STOP driving when that little inner voice, or your grown child, tells you you're not safe (nor is the public) to drive anymore. If you insist that you must have that wheel in your hands, go out in an open field and have a ball! But ask the farmer—and the bull—for permission first!

Two dear old friends took turns every Sunday driving around town where they had grown up. As they were cruising along, they came to an intersection. Although the light turned red, they rolled right on through. The passenger thought to herself, "Well, it must have been safe, I suppose."

At the very next light, the exact same thing happened, only this time they had a narrow miss with another car! The passenger was sure they were in the wrong but wasn't certain what to say.

At the very next intersection, the light was red even before they got to it, but her friend drove right through again, just as she had the other two. This time the woman in the passenger seat had had enough. "Stella, you just ran three red lights in a row! You could have killed us both!"

Stella turned to her and said, "Oh, my! Am I driving?" (*Old Jokes for Old Folks*. This was a favorite of mine and my mother's when we were driving somewhere.)

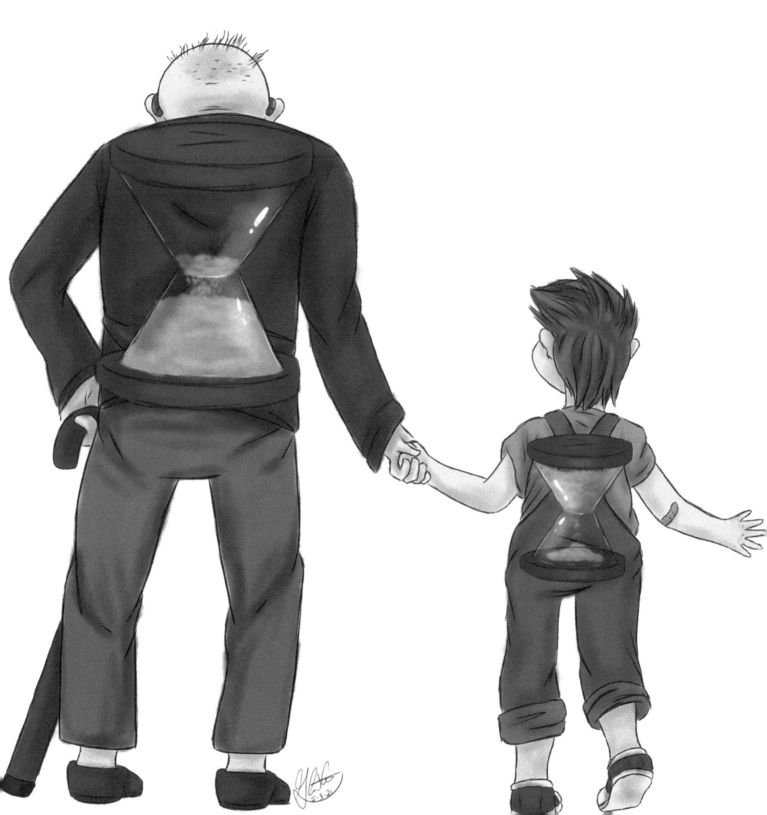

Mind

Don't mess with OLD PEOPLE. We didn't get this age by BEING STUPID! (Facebook)

One minute, you're young and fun. And the next, you're turning down the stereo in your car to see better. (Facebook)

Life's tragedy is that we get OLD too soon and WISE too late. (Benjamin Franklin, Founding Father of the United States)

Now, people live from day to day, but they do not count the time.
They don't see the days slipping by and neither do I.
(James Taylor, American singer/songwriter, "Anywhere but Heaven")

Do you remember Burma-Shave signs? They certainly saved a boring trip or two! BUT if you do, it is a dead giveaway for your age. The signs appeared for 37 years from 1926 to 1963 (*Wikipedia*). Just to bring a grin:

When crossing intersections, Look each way. A harp sounds nice, But it's hard to play. Burma Shave.

Do the best you can until you know better.
Then when you know better, do better.
(Maya Angelou, American poet)

Every time an old person dies, it's like a library burning down. (Alex Haley, American writer)

My, how I felt this way when Mother died! She contained a WEALTH of information that I can no longer easily access...and I miss that.
When someone you love becomes a memory, that memory becomes a treasure.

Sometimes I wish I could just rewind back to the old days with my loved ones and press pause...just for a little while. (Facebook)

Tradition—peer pressure from dead people. (Facebook)

Everything will be all right in the end. If it is not all right, it is not the end.

(*Head jerk*) AAAARRRRGHHH—what you feel when a professional person in the room says something about her dad...and you realize she's speaking of a MUCH younger person than you! Or that, God forbid, her GRANDPARENTS are your age or younger!

I want you to think about your parents for a moment. Your birthday is their celebration. Your happiness is their joy. Your future is their legacy. If they had to bury you, it would kill them. So please, next time they say, "Be safe" or "Let me know you get there, okay," don't just brush it off because, to them, you are everything. (Facebook)

Birthdays should celebrate YOUR MOTHER as much as they celebrate you! After all, she was there too!

Children are the rainbow of life.
Grandchildren are the pot of gold.

Doorways wipe out memory. (Barbara, age 67; writer's note—pretty profound)

I hate when I put something in a "safe place" and then it's pretty much safe forever.

I'm old enough to make my own decisions...just not young enough to remember what I decided. (Facebook)

HAPPY BIRTHDAY! Just remember one thing...
And you'll be doing really well!

My birthday present to you—whenever you start forgetting stuff and sounding confused and crazy (which you have been for many, many years), I promise to tell everyone you're drunk so they don't think it's because you're old. (Charlie, age 68; writer's note—Thank you very much for the present, Charles! I'll have you know **I'm** 66 for the third time.)

Vignette

Charlie is a CPA and spent most of his career as corporate comptroller of the **Ogden Newspapers Inc.** of Wheeling, West Virginia. A right GENIUS individual, I figure, no thanks to me. We attended all but 2 years of our formal education together, most of it with me right behind him due to the alphabetical order of our names, which dictated seating. In grade school, I spent my time breaking pencils over his head when I needed help; I locked him in the stage storage with "a friend" in high school. But the best of all was helping his college roommates make purple Kool-Aid in the toilet on a party weekend in Morgantown, West Virginia (WVU, the party school winner for years), and giving it to him as Purple Jesus, a famous poor college student imbibement of the era consisting of grape Kool-Aid and grain alcohol. Then they showed him the toilet "where they'd made it." HYSTERICAL! (We disagree on some of these details, but it nevertheless turned out pretty well. Despite all of this, we have been dear friends for more than 60 years and tend to stick to fun-making birthday cards to each other now. Yes, I'm older by only 3 months!)

When you're young, you think everyone older than you knows everything; but when it's you, you understand that basically everyone is winging it and doesn't really have their life together just like you. (Sloan, age 24)

Don't worry about getting older. You're still gonna do dumb stuff, only slower. (Facebook)

The older I get, the dumber I realize everyone else is.

I'm a lot smarter than I used to be, but I'm still dumb. I can still put my foot in my mouth. (Dr. Tim, age 42)

When is this "old enough to know better" supposed to kick in? (Facebook)

When did my WILD OATS turn into SHREDDED WHEAT?

As life unfolds, you get wiser and more grounded. (Fran Drescher, American actor, "Taking Back My Life," *People* magazine, February 17, 2020; writer's note—Really? I'm waiting...)

Reread your favorite book at different stages of your life. The plot never changes, but your perspective does. (Facebook)

Prepare for retirement starting at a young age. (Debbie from Old Navy)

According to the U.S. Bureau of Labor Statistics, about half of small business employees do not have access to the same quality work-based retirement plans as workers at large employers...largely due to cost restraints. However, a new law, the Setting Every Community Up for Retirement Enhancement (SECURE) Act, allows small businesses to pool their resources to offer retirement plans to workers that are cost

efficient and easier to administer thereby providing more secure retire-
ment environments for employees. (Steve Bulger, acting administrator,
Mid-Atlantic Region, US Small Business Administration, "Act Benefits,"
Cumberland Times-News, January 27, 2020, editorial page 4A)

Since COVID hit shortly after this article was released, the status of this act may
have been disrupted, as have small businesses. It's still worth checking into as an employer
and as an employee.

> Retirement must be wonderful. I mean, you can suck in your stomach
> for only so long. (Burt Reynolds, American actor)

I had a creepy kind of feeling in Florida when I looked around, and I was surrounded
by OLD people AS FAR AS THE EYE COULD SEE! I couldn't believe how old people my age are.

SUNDOWNERS. I'd never heard of it.

> It occurs with older people in the late afternoons or early evenings.
> They may become depressed because they think they're approaching the
> end of their lives—kind of like seeing the light at the end of their tunnel.
> They're not sure where they are or what they're supposed to do, EVERY
> DAY! (Noni, pharmacy tech, age 63)

> Rapidly shrinking brain is how a doctor described it. I wouldn't wish
> DEMENTIA or ALZHEIMER'S on anyone. As the patient's brain slowly dies,
> they change physically and eventually forget who their loved ones are.
> Patients can eventually become bedridden, unable to move, and unable to
> eat or drink. (Facebook)

When Dad started showing signs of **dementia**, we needed to scurry to U̲N̲hide weap-
ons from him (he had hidden his guns to keep them away from his young grandson, and it
was West Virginia; we have always had guns for shooting varmints and vittles but not for

shooting each other)! But we didn't know what spaces he'd stuffed them in. However, his now-adult grandson knew from childhood where he'd hidden them.

Common signs and symptoms of **dementia** *(from the MAYO CLINIC)*

Cognitive changes

— Memory loss, usually noticed by someone else (I mean, how do you know you forgot it if you didn't remember in the first place?)
— Difficulty communicating or finding the right words
— Getting lost going someplace familiar

When my dad was in the early stages of dementia and before we were sure what was happening, we went boating with him in the 1000 Islands in Canada, like we had for years. As usual, he went charging in and around the many islands, which was a bit tricky sometimes if you didn't know your way, which he always had. When we got to the wide openness of 30 Acres—named that because there are no islands, just open water—he stopped the boat, looked around, and announced, "I don't know where I am." It was absolutely the WORST place this could happen because the rest of us hadn't paid any attention to our route, because Dad was THE CAPTAIN!

I don't remember now how we limped lamely back to the cottage, but we were onto him then.

— Difficulty with problem-solving
— Difficulty handling complex tasks

Warning—the beginning of dementia can lead to leaving the tractor running while getting off to pick wildflowers, only to find that said tractor had taken itself by the wheel and driven down the hill and crashed over the bank into a pile of parts behind the barn. Trust me. I know these things. NO, it wasn't me!

— Difficulty planning and organizing

— Difficulty with coordination and motor functions
— Confusion and disorientation

Psychological changes

— Personality changes
— Depression
— Anxiety
— Inappropriate behavior

I once turned around at a Lions Club picnic and found myself staring at one of the members relieving himself...out in broad daylight...right there by the road not 8 feet away from me. Thank GOD he was facing the other way. Within a year or 2, he had a diagnosis of dementia, but not before he entertained others with assorted other behaviors.

— Paranoia
— Agitation
— Hallucinations

Check with your doctor if you see these things happening in those close to you or if others note these things relative to you.

YEARS ago, I went through an extensive battery of tests for **Alzheimer's** because I was having memory issues. Thank GOD it was determined that I did not have it. However, that nagging term kept running through my mind; so the next visit that I had with my family physician, I asked him about it too. His retort was something like this, "If you forget something and it comes back to you, it's not Alzheimer's." That sounded pretty helpful and hopeful. However, it occurred to me that, if you forgot something, you wouldn't know you forgot it, would you?

There is a difference between forgetfulness and dementia. However, apparently, it's an accepted fact that people, as they age, don't remember things as well. For example, when I went to the hospital for a test recently, I registered, stopped at the bathroom—

okay, restroom—gathered my purse, and went for my test. At the desk, the lady asked me if I had some paperwork to give her. Looking at my empty hands, I told her no, so she proceeded to generate the documents I needed for the test. All was well. However, when I went back to the hospital a couple of days later, one of my friends up there practically rolled on the floor as she recounted another patient discovering my papers in the restroom. She knew full well that I had forgotten all about them. BUT I DID remember them then and the lady at the window popping out the stickers and putting my wrist label on me, the one that was on me when I said I'd gotten no papers. It all goes TOGETHER! Guess it wasn't dementia!

YOUNG WITCH: Eye of newt, belladonna, hair of bat, arsenic, tail of werewolf, blood of a virgin.

WITCH, 50-PLUS: Oh, crap, forgot the ingredients. Oh, ya…vodka, Xanax, ginko biloba, calcium, estrogen, chocolate, coffee, and hair of Sam Elliot. (Facebook)

Let's think about this remembery thing, particularly if you live alone and are responsible for all of the house and car and EVERYTHING! It would serve you well to get an inexpensive calendar or planner and put all those important dates in there—like car inspections and tags, insurance annual or semiannual payments, bills paid only once a year, and tax day (and a cue several weeks before that you need to have all your papers gathered up and prepared)—and put it where you can find it, NOT SOMEWHERE WHERE "YOU WON'T LOSE IT," because you know THAT stuff **always** gets lost! Oh, and get in a habit of checking every day to see what the day and date are, especially if you live alone. You can do this on your phone, computer, calendar, TV, and other resources. As we've isolated ourselves during this COVID-19 time, I've found myself needing to check these things because we're not going out and there are no activity reference points, like church on Sunday for United Methodists.

Best doormat EVER (and place it so it faces you as YOU GO OUT the door):

> Did you remember?
> Keys
> Wallet
> Phone

I pray I don't get Alzheimer's. (Jennifer, hairstylist, age 37, who's been there/done that with her grandmother)

From WebMD, these are the 10 early signs of Alzheimer's:

1. Memory loss
2. Trouble planning and problem-solving
3. Daily tasks are a challenge
4. Times and places are confusing
5. Changes in vision
6. Words and conversations are frustrating
7. You lose things
8. Lapse in judgment
9. Social withdrawal
10. Mood changes

Heck, my family won't notice the difference in me. I already exhibit half of these! You can guess which ones.

From Leezo's Care Connection, Hospice Care of the Southwest,_Alzheimer's communication:

1. Never ARGUE, instead AGREE.
2. Never REASON, instead DIVERT.
3. Never SHAME, instead DISTRACT.
4. Never LECTURE, REASSURE.
5. Never say, "REMEMBER," instead REMINISCE.

6. Never say, "I TOLD YOU," instead REPEAT/REGROUP.
7. Never say, "YOU CAN'T," instead do what you CAN.
8. Never COMMAND/DEMAND, instead ASK/MODEL.
9. Never CONDESCEND, instead ENCOURAGE.
10. Never FORCE, REINFORCE.

The transition comes slowly, as it began between her and her mother. The changing of power. The transferring of responsibility. The passing down of duty. Suddenly, you are spewing out the familiar phrases learned at the knee of your mother.

"Of course, you're sick. Don't you think I know when you're not feeling well?"

"So, where's your sweater?"

"Do you have to go to the bathroom before we go?"

But slowly and insidiously and certainly the years give way and there is no one to turn to... The daughter comtemplates, "It wasn't supposed to be this way. All the years I was bathed, dressed, fed, advised disciplined, ordered, cared for and had every need anticipated, I wanted my turn to come when I could command. Now that it's here, why am I so sad?" (Erma Bombeck, GREAT American author, *if life is a bowl of cherries, what am I doing in the pits*?)

Hindsight may be 20/20, but nobody's perfect. We make mistakes. We say wrong things. We do wrong things. We fall. We get up. We learn. We grow. We move and we live! (Facebook)

Remember, children, as you gallantly move your aging parents in with you, they've left their friends at THEIR homes. They will miss them and still need them. Sometimes those friends are even their "chosen" family, no slight to you, of course.

WHEN PARENTS GET OLD,

Let them grow old with the same love that they let you grow. Let them speak and tell repeated stories with the same patience and interest that they heard yours as a child. Let them overcome, like so many times when they let you win. Let them enjoy their friends just as they let you. Let them enjoy the talks with their grandchildren because they see you in them. Let them enjoy living among the objects that have accompanied them for a long time because they suffer when they feel that you tear pieces of this life away. Let them be wrong, like so many times you have been wrong and they didn't embarrass you by correcting you. LET THEM LIVE and try to make them happy the last stretch of the path they have left to go; give them your hand, just like they gave you their hand when you started your path!
(Deacon Karl Koberger, St. Joseph Catholic Church, Gulfport, Mississippi, via Facebook)

Honor your mother and father and your days shall be long upon the earth. (God)

One good thing about aging is no schedules—go to bed or get up whenever you want. For the most part, your time is your time until all the doctors start with all the appointments for all the aches and pains that start with age. You can stay up all night watching movies you may have seen before, but you don't always remember seeing them or at least part of them. I have more negatives than positive things about aging. You don't have much "housework" (the writer: and that's a negative?) to do, but it takes longer to do it. You don't need to worry about wearing out your clothes or shoes because you've been collecting them for a long time. The best thing about aging is grandkids. They are way more fun than your own kids. I guess, since you have more time and money, there's less stress with grandkids. You get to cuddle, spoil, and love the heck out of them; then give them back to their parents. I get lots of exercise because of forgetting what I got up to get. I also like not worrying about what other people think or taking bullcrap from them. I also feel closer to friends. I may have less friends, but they are better friends. You really know who you can trust and depend on. I'm also happy to still be breathing and able to move and get around, maybe slower, but still getting around and enjoying life more. (Stella, retired teacher, age 73)

The importance of **HOBBIES**: a friend says developing and/or researching a hobby is imperative. She has taught herself computer usage and enhanced that to reading on her Kindle through the West Virginia Library Commission's HOOPLA. She reads to her husband about history and politics. They watch *Jeopardy* and TURNER classic movies. She sews, knits, and gardens, even overwintering a Mandevilla, which is not native to our area.

Although her husband has limited use of the computer due to arthritis, he loves to read Civil War, WWI, and WWII history; Bible devotionals; *Packard* magazines; and the local newspapers.

Together they do a weekly tour of the farm after church and are interested in the goings-on in both. They even have four sheep they tend. They believe in teamwork. She's adamant about hobbies because she saw her mother work so hard on the farm, and when her body wore out, she had nothing to fall back on. (Pat and Charles, both age 88)

Beware of the lasting effects of watching the BEE GEES, three of them, on PBS in their final concert or any of our long-ago favorites possibly. For days after that evening, I was profoundly depressed. Was it because they are all gone now but Barry or that I'll never have a chance to meet them (like I ever would have)? My brain just could not compute.

However, hearing old music you used to love is like getting in touch with an old friend. (Facebook)

What's a Will? It is <u>not</u> the same thing as a living will.
The answer is a dead giveaway. (Pastor Roy; remember him?)

Seriously, do your will LONG before you anticipate needing it! If you do not know what to do about that, see a lawyer or look online...but DO

IT! As you age or become infirmed, consider putting all of your property into someone else's name, like your kids', who are due to inherit it anyway. Otherwise, your hard-earned savings for your children will be sucked up in nursing home fees. Or you could become an incredible burden (even though they'll lovingly do it) on your family, who don't want to see all those assets go up in smoke. (Uli, teacher, age 62)

There are attorneys who specialize in elder law and can help you put your will together.

The worst parts of getting older:
— Living alone
— Doing for myself whether I want to or not
— Learning patience
(Myrtle, age 94)

Vignette

Myrtle is one of my nonagenarian friends. Having attended a thought-provoking class together for several years, our spirits are so aligned that age has faded away, and I wonder sometimes why she won't do some things anymore. However, when a certain questionable 3 book series came out, we could be caught exchanging small brown paper bags... in church...and giggling!
And then there's TIME.

You know you're getting older when you open a fortune cookie and your fortune has a "use by" date. (*Old Jokes for Old Folks*)

Time is precious. Don't waste it. (Facebook)

I had a church acquaintance who told me she'd always wanted to dye her dark hair red after she saw mine. I told her I would even help her, but she sadly went to her grave never having taken the time.

Most of us spend our time neatly tucked away, all safe and sound in our tidy little lives. Almost without our noticing, the days start to take on a shade of gray. It's not that we don't long for a change... It's just that sometimes we get so busy that we forget how to really live! Busting loose and abandoning our fears is easier said than done. To willingly leave the safety of our comfort zone and reach into the fire requires a huge leap of faith. But just on the other side, far beyond our wildest imagination, is a magical, mystical, uncharted territory called POSSIBILITY. (Suzy Toronto, *Life Is All about How You Handle Plan B*)

Amazingly, one of my physicians, Dr. Neil Crowe, age 63, related a phenomenon which helps to explain the feeling of time passing more quickly as we age. He opines:

Our perception of time is very much based on a subconscious comparison with our total life experience. As a child, having lived only a very few years, a few weeks is a relatively large percentage of the child's life. For this reason, this seems like a very long time compared with the child's subconscious time base.

However, as we age, a few weeks is a relative pittance of time when compared with the total amount of time we have socked away in our subconscious memory. Thus, those few weeks just seem to flit by.

An analogy could be a car trip. If one is driving across town, a 20-mile additional journey would add quite a bit to the trip and would seem quite long.

If one is completing a transcontinental journey, an additional 20 miles would be perceived as a very short little jaunt.

It takes longer to do things, like getting ready to go somewhere. Allow for that. I do. I'm always late anyway. Someone has to be last; I just volunteer for it. I could always say, "Sorry I'm late. I got here as soon as I wanted to." But I DIDN'T when the young upstarts at the hair salon chastised me for being a tad—okay, 15 minutes—late.

Thirty years goes a lot faster than you think it does. (Mark Calaway, a.k.a. The Undertaker, American retired professional wrestler in WWE, *People*, November 30, 2020)

Sixty seconds now feels more like thirty
Tick-tock, won't stop, around it goes
Sand through the glass sure falls in a hurry
And all you keep trying to do is slow it down, soak it in
Keep trying to make the good times last as long as you can
But you can't, yeah, man
It goes too fast
It's just goes too fast
Way too fast.
(**Luke Bryan**, American singer/songwriter, "Fast")

How fast things can happen! 6 kids, 2nd husband, 3 knee surgeries, and two carpal tunnels and 4 brain cells left. Just not ready for any of it! (Stephanie, only age 42)

If I had it to do over, I wouldn't have married so young and would have traveled. Because I was young with 6 children close together, and I couldn't travel. (Robbie, artist, age 82)

Travel. Do things you've always wanted to do! There's not going to be any better time than the present. So you didn't get to do something when you were younger; do it NOW! I have a friend who wants to go skydiving for her 70th birthday (it's somehow almost her 73rd). Guess she wants to copy President George H. W. Bush, who went skydiving every 5th birthday after his retirement!

You see, it's not surprising that some people wait till they're 80 to take up skydiving. If you're going to have your life flash before your eyes, at least it will be a longer trip. (*Old Jokes for Old Folks*)

I've watched too many people delay travel and adventure with the idea that they will enjoy those things in retirement, only to have those plans disrupted by illness or other life demands. Don't delay all of your travel and adventures and assume you'll get the chance later. If you have the time and money to do something you want to do, do it now! (Ian, age 39)

Vignette

Ian is my son, a public relations senior vice president, who is usually quite remarkable. When I needed his thoughts on aging to fill in his age group (which he's less than a year of changing dramatically), his introspective comments took me aback. He doesn't view his (or my) aging very hopefully. For 3 weeks at least in the beginning of the COVID-19 pandemic, he managed to scare the beejeebers out of me with reminders that I'm in "that age group" and I have "health issues." I have NEVER felt so close to kicking the bucket in my life! I usually feel like I'm closer to his age, hence the 40-year disappearing act.

Speaking of travel, just keep in mind the accessibility of the trip if you have any issues. Some cruise ships do not accommodate wheelchairs, but you can be wheeled through airports by contacting their accessibility office. These $5 tip rides have given me the opportunity to take several flights following surgery or injuries. I hate to have someone else do things like that for me, but then I remind myself that this is THEIR livelihood. The same applies for porters in airports (and hotels.) They will load those heavy suitcases...and golf clubs...and carry-ons onto their carts with magical balancing skill and be unloading them at check-in before you can finish printing your boarding passes! Isn't that well worth a $5 or $10 tip depending on the distance and amount of assistance? Don't go if you can't afford your tips! Oh, and most trains between gates have priority seating for those who don't feel like taking the risk of standing.

As one ages, so does the energy supply. You may find that you have more energy in the morning, and you just poop out by afternoon. Wonder if that's why soap operas were invented?

I'm a person who wants to do a lot of things trapped in a body that doesn't. (Recipes for the Family, Facebook)

By the time you age into having "a lot of it," either you're in the empty-nest period when the kids aren't there anymore to use it on, or you're just retired and in the don't-know-what-to-get-into stage or you're into the lonely nobody-comes-to-visit years. Join groups for your own enjoyment or to help others. Doing for others is a proven mood booster for the person doing the helping! Keep in mind that, although you may not be able to get out and physically help someone, you can provide support via the phone or the internet! My mother and I had this discussion more than once when she'd feel a little down. Form your own support group with people whose needs and characteristics are similar to yours. My Facebook Messenger group, bless their hearts, understand me no matter how abstract I may be, which probably may mean they're a little abstract themselves! So we support one another, joke together, and care about each other. A few words from somebody who remembered you can mean a lot, like, "You'd better tuck your crazy back in. It's starting to show." (Honest to gosh, that was one of the things!)

Then perhaps you will have made enough friends that loneliness won't be such a sad problem for you. Just ask any worker like Glenna, my illustrator, or visitor in an adult-care facility how sad it is to see residents who never have any visitors...day after day, month after month. If you're a relative, shame on you! If you're a friend, you're gonna be there, maybe not once a week, but once in a while at least!

I used to tell my students to remember me in my old age...and I MEANT it! Poor kids.

Respect those who rode the trail before you because...someday, sooner than you imagine, you'll be old too. (Facebook)

Your cell phone has already replaced your watch, camera, calendar, and alarm clock. Don't let it replace your family. (Facebook)

Sadness warning. An old man took his phone to a repair shop.
Repairer said, "Nothing is wrong with this phone."
Old man, with tears in his eyes, said, "Then why don't my children ever call me?" (Facebook)

Dear Abby:

This is a message about our senior population. Our children grow up, marry and have children. Each grandchild is special. We love them. Then the grandkids grow up and have little ones of their own. By this time we're old and sometimes need help with housework, yard work, or just would like to get out of the house to go eat or shop. We still have feelings, and we're not dead. But while it may not be intentional, it seems there is no time for the elderly.

We may say we're fine and don't mind being alone, but it IS lonely at times. No one calls to say hello or ask if we need anything. How long does it take to make a call? It would be nice if each family member called once a week or came by once a month. The love we've always had for family is still there and strong.

Children and grandchildren, please think about this and remember: The most important thing you can give your elderly relatives is your TIME. Time is the most precious gift of all and doesn't cost a thing. Someday you will be old, too.

—Wise Woman in North Carolina
(Dear Abby, a syndicated column, Facebook)

While there're many differences between Korean and Vietnamese, my culture (Vietnamese) is like many around the world, not just Asian but also Latino and even some European, who have the utmost respect for elders. Families live together or very closely. There is no separation. When it comes to their golden years, the family knits together to give care and take them in. The filial duty to parents is how we are raised, and it's commonly discussed how sad it is that Americans send their elders away to nursing homes. My grandma currently lives with my uncle. We are excited to be reunited this July and celebrate her 90th birthday.

This reverence for elder generations, family heritage, and time-honored traditions is also why it's so incredibly painful and gut wrenching that our elders are being murdered and attacked by racist bigots in this country who don't understand what it means to be foreigners, different, or feel less than because you look different or sound different. (Evan, age 41) (writer's note—this is so very painful for me to hear because we love Evan so dearly)

I questioned Evan after a visit with another friend, Cliff, who, when I mentioned this book, related that it had been an odd topic of discussion in his family. His mother is Korean, and his father was American. It made their heads spin at the difference in viewpoint on elder care. Just as Evan stated, the Asian communities embrace and care for their elderly while the White (?) societies put their elderly in care facilities away from the families for whom they had so dearly loved and cared. Please tuck back in my White privilege. It's showing and just had its head jerked again with realization.

Discussion overheard between Kenny and our good friend:
"Why does it seem like so many more people are dying?"
"Because, as we get older, we have accumulated friends for years. Then, when they start dying off, it just seems to be so many," Diana, age 72, said.
"We're getting closer!" Kenny, age 76, replied.

We know that older Americans are at greater risk for SOCIAL ISO-LATION, which can lead to physical illness, depression, and even dementia. But scientists now say there are medical causes—and remedies—for this painful condition that affects more of us each year. (Lynn Darling, *AARP the Magazine*, December 2019 / January 2020)

From Ms. Darling's article also came this information. According to Louise Hawkley, a senior research scientist at the University of Chicago, "There is a human need to be embedded, connected, integrated in a social network." When that social network is missing, "the consequences are very real in terms of mental and physical health." Continuing from Ms. Darling,

Loneliness is a killer—an array of studies have found that it leaves us more likely to die from heart disease and is a contributing factor in other fatal conditions. It makes us more vulnerable to Alzheimer's disease, high blood pressure, suicide, even the common cold.

And this will shock you, continuing from the AARP report, **"It's more dangerous to our health, researchers tell us, than obesity, and it's the equivalent to smoking 15 cigarettes a day."**

Data is showing that we are tending more toward social isolation. More people are living alone (there is a 32 percent higher risk of early death for those living alone). Fewer are married, and fewer have children. There is a stigma regarding loneliness to the point that applying the term social connection may be more user-friendly. Plus, embedded in the loneliness are feelings of rejection, disconnection, and longing that produce pain as real as physical injury, which may actually result in inflammation and may damage the immune system. Through a complex dance of systems interacting, "the brain becomes irritable, suspicious, prone to negative emotions, and fearful of meeting new people and making new friends." It may lead to a distorted reality of the world around them. So what the person desperately needs may be the very thing the brain does not agree on. Therefore, throwing 2 lonely people together, which would have been my bright idea, would be exactly the wrong thing. Sometimes it takes therapy to break down these misconceptions by the brain. And perhaps some ALEVE for the inflammation, the article suggested.

There is some exploration into the use of virtual reality to stave off isolation. "Watch this space," as Rachel Maddow would say.

> When a community does something together, that community is very happy, jovial, connected, and unified. (Larry P. Aiken, CHIPPEWA)

> "All she needed was a listener...no advice, wisdom, experience, money, assistance, expertise or even compassion...but just a minute or two to listen." (Erma Bombeck, *if life is a bowl of cherries, what am i doing in the pits?*)

Quit saying, "I should go see [somebody]," but you don't go. Eventually you may not have that option.

We don't stop playing because we grow old; we grow old because we stop playing.

If they don't exist already, set up programs in your community to pair "seniors" with kids, ones who could also use the companionship, or help with homework. That bit of young energy, in moderation, certainly couldn't hurt. We're letting a lot of valuable resources go down the tubes by not putting bored older folks and kids together! BTW, there are also a lot of kids, either ignored or damaged by drug environments, who would benefit from a secure person. I realize there could be issues with liability, but where there's a will, there's a way if it's important.

Or come up with an idea out of the box, like offering to go to the hospital to rock babies who are going through withdrawal thanks to their mom's drug use. We are in a drug crisis. There probably are a lot of them unfortunately. Children are taking a huge hit from this epidemic.

> *Si, se puede*, Spanish for "Yes, we can." Every moment is an organizing opportunity, every person a potential activist, every minute a chance to change the world. (Dolores Huerta, advocate for workers, immigrants, children, and women)

> Researchers have found that people who are socially connected live longer. And those who have community outreach keeping an eye on them and including them, be it the mailman or the hairdresser, do better. We've known that in small communities for years. It's just a matter of people stepping out of their own little worlds and paying attention. [Writer's note—Okay, I can hear it now. This is NOT sticking your nose in somebody else's business. It's just providing a little support.] (Lynn Darling, "Is There a Cure for Loneliness?" *AARP the Magazine*, December 2019 / January 2020)

This brings me to a chuckle, especially after grinding through that other stuff.

A 95-year-young lady at church, carrying 2 bowls of soup and her oxygen tank, was asked if she needed help. I understand now that that may have been a mistake. She replied tartly, "Why? Do I look like I need help?" And on her merry way she went!

You think suicide is cowardly? I'll tell you what's cowardly. Hurting someone so much that they want to end their lives. (Facebook)

Although this is often the case for suicide, this is not the whole story for seniors. This is from "Elder Suicide: The Risks, Detection, and How to Help," **AgingInPlace. org**, February 2020:

Suicide rates have increased by more than 30% since 1999 in the United States, according to the Centers for Disease Control and Prevention (CDC). Males have a higher rate than females. Additionally, this risk increases with age: 75- to 85-year-olds having higher rates of suicide than those who are between 65 and 75, and individuals 85 or older have the highest risk yet. [Now, these numbers took me aback.] The second most commonly reported cause of suicide is experiencing a life crisis within the previous two weeks.

Factors that seem to lead to this choice are relationship issues, experiencing a life crisis, substance abuse (i.e., alcohol), physical health issues, employment and/or financial factors, legal issues, housing-related stress, and isolation.

Early suicide warning signs:

— Person expresses depression or hopelessness
— There's been a loss of independence
— Diagnosis of a serious medical condition that could shorten life
— Social isolation
— Recent death of loved one or family issues
— Lack of ability to or desire to deal with change
— Demonstration of risky behaviors
— Substance use or abuse has increased
— Previous suicide attempt or statements that the world would be better off without them
— Unusual giving away of personal possessions

Suicide prevention options for seniors:

— Talk with them nonjudgmentally about options for positive activities.
— Connect them with elderly support groups.
— Limit access to substances and lethal means.

Cheer up! These guys prove living with others is beneficial.

Three brothers—age 92, 94, and 96—live in a house together.

One night, the 96-year-old draws a bath, puts his foot in, and pauses. He yells down the stairs, "Was I getting in or out of the bath?"

The 94-year-old yells back, "I don't know. I'll come up and see." He starts up the stairs and pauses, then he yells, "Was I going up the stairs or coming down?"

The 92-year-old was sitting at the kitchen table having coffee, listening to his brothers. He shakes his head and says, "I sure hope I never get that forgetful." He knocks on wood for good luck. He then yells, "I'll come up and help both of you as soon as I see who's at the door." (Facebook)

Guard against SCAMS ALL THE TIME AT EVERY AGE! We all know that the nuisance calls with funny numbers that ring from dawn to dusk ARE scams. **Do not give out any personal info over the phone** even if you're told that they are the IRS, USPS, UPS, or GOD! Don't do it unless they have some **foolproof** method of confirming who they are. And don't let them scare you in the middle night with a call from your "grandson who is in jail and needs money to get out" (delivered with a lot of whining, begging, crying, and whatever else they think will work). This ruse scared my mother for years until the phone company assured her this guy had been caught. See, in the back of her mind was this worry still that it might have been her grandson. Nighttime fog can do that. However, even in bright daylight, a call from the "IRS" can scare the beejeebers out of you. Just **don't give them any information.** The real IRS will not call you by phone!

A cyber security tip I heard recently was to not be caught up in computer programs that say "You've got a problem with your computer" and that you need to follow their directions, which include letting them take over your computer and remotely control it. All kinds of bad things can, and do (don't ask how; I know this for sure), happen, like being billed ungodly amounts with no way to track the scammers. No matter how entertaining it is to see your computer controlled in a ghostly way, it's not worth the risk. I'm here to tell you! DON'T ASK!

And it will likely come at some point, Younger Ones, that you will have to take over for your parents; and it may not be pleasant. But it is a necessary evil as decision-making skills decline in the older years. And it's another good reason to travel BEFORE you retire and may be needed at home.

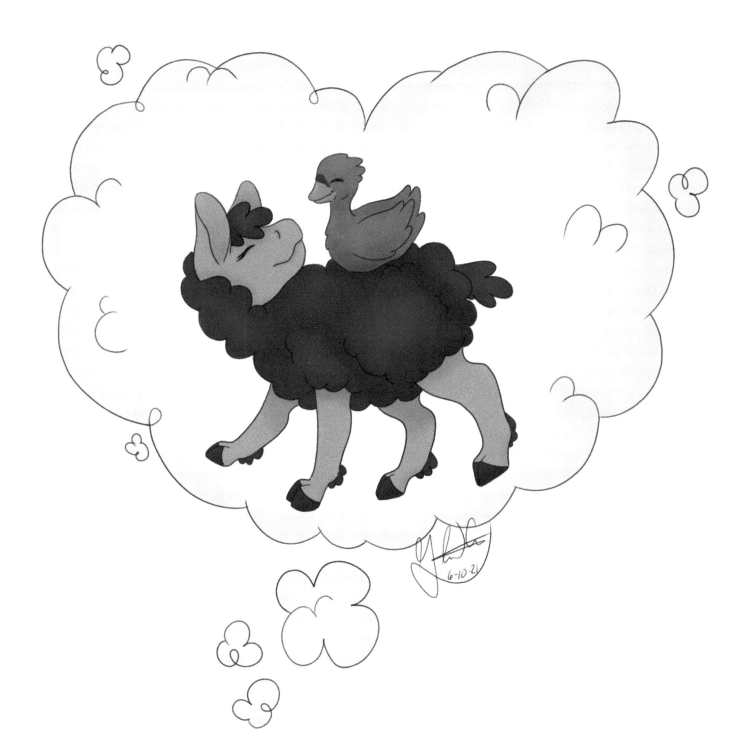

Attitude

(Section Suggested by Lisa, Therapist, Age 58)

If you're lucky enough to get old, you should celebrate it. What's wrong with being 72 or 82 or 92? If God is good enough to give you those years, flaunt them. (Iris Apfel, American businesswoman, interior designer, nonagenarian, and fashion icon, age 98, "You'll see the Light," *Hemispheres* magazine, January 2020)

THE OLDER YOU GET, the more you realize it is okay to live a life others don't understand. (Facebook)

I like weird people. The black sheep, the odd ducks, the rejects, the loners, the lost, and forgotten.
More often than not, these people have the most beautiful souls. (Facebook; writer's note—but it could've come from me)

At the end of the day, I'd rather be excluded for who I include than for who I exclude. (Facebook)

While chatting with someone at the beauty parlor / hair salon / whatever, we stumbled onto the name of a friend we had in common. I hadn't thought about Nell in years. Way into her 90s, she was still "taking" her exercises. She told me about teaching lipreading long ago at the West Virginia School for the Deaf when sign language was forbidden. Talk about beating your head against a brick wall! Have you ever tried to understand what's being said on TV when the volume's turned off? ANYWAY, as I understand it, she also hung her car in a tree and was dangling from the seat belt when they found her. What a cackle she had over that one! THAT'S the kind of character I want to be!

Be the kind of aging person that, when your feet hit the floor in the morning, the devil says, "O crap! She's up!"

Truth is powerful, and it prevails. (Sojourner Truth, who gained her freedom in 1827, was an African American abolitionist and women's rights activist, "Ain't I a Woman?" speech, May 9, 1851)

Strong women aren't simply born. They are made by the storms they walk through. (Facebook)

Strong women don't have attitudes. They have standards and boundaries. (Facebook)

I'd Pick More Daisies

If I had my life to live over, I'd try to make more mistakes next time. I would relax, I would limber up. I would be simpler than I have been this trip. I would take more trips. I would climb more mountains and swim more rivers. I would eat more ice cream and less bran. I would have more actual troubles and fewer imaginary ones.

You see, I am one of those maidens who live prophylactically and sensibly and sanely, hour after hour, and if I had it to do over again, I'd have more of them. In fact, I'd try to have nothing else. Just moments one after another, instead of living so many years ahead each day. I have been one of those persons who never goes anywhere without a thermometer, a raincoat and a parachute.

If I had my life to live over, I would start barefoot earlier in the spring and stay that way later in the fall. I would play hooky more. I wouldn't make such good grades except by accident. I would have more dogs. I would have more sweethearts, drink more tomato juice. I would go to more dances, and ride on more merry-go-rounds, I'd pick more daisies. (**Chatterbox**, Sunnyside Van Ness Convalescent Hospital, July 1979)

Being old is like being a dog. The high points of the day are scratching, peeing, and watching for the mailman. (*Old Jokes for Old Folks*)

When I asked my 97-year-young friend Jewell about aging, she said, "Laugh a lot. Better keep in touch with God. Keep being myself."

Vignette

Okay, so Jewell's not quite right. Neither am I. But we've liked each other this way for about 40 years!

She is one of my older friends, but it's not a stuffy, patronizing relationship. We have ornery streaks, which haven't gone away with age, unless we get too stuffy. We love hoohaaing over the same things. LONG ago, she showed me a kindness that I've never forgotten. Oh, and we may have snickered together in church a couple of times before that.

I didn't grow up poor. I grew up rich with things money could never buy. We always had lots of love, we were taught to respect our elders, and we learned about good work ethic. Our greatest riches were our family and our faith in God. (Shelby Condo, Kelly's Treehouse)

If you want to change the world, go home and love your family. (Mother Teresa, Roman Catholic nun and missionary)

Irish diplomacy—the art of telling someone to go to hell and having them look forward to the trip!

You're never too old to set another goal or to dream new dreams. (C. S. Lewis, writer)

The goal is to die with memories not dreams. (Facebook)

Don't stop learning and growing no matter your age. Probably the most dangerous phrase that anyone could use in the world today is that dreadful one: "BUT WE'VE ALWAYS DONE IT THAT WAY." Every aging person should have a mentor of the younger group to keep them in touch with current reality, fashion trends, technology, and that sort of thing so being stuck in the rut like this does not occur. Glenna, Darrah, Aisa, and Reggae help me out.

If you're over 45 and don't have an under-30 mentor-not mentee-mentor, then you're going to miss fundamental shifts in thinking that are happening. (Facebook) My goodness, do I miss this! I think I aged 20 years when I retired and no longer had my students to keep me up on things; I didn't know which emojis were for what or the songs that were current...and what they said/meant, or drug names...

You may shoot me with your words. You may cut me with your eyes. You may kill me with your hatefulness, BUT STILL, LIKE AIR, I'LL RISE. (Maya Angelou, award-winning poet, actress, dancer, writer, and civil rights leader)

Bullying is not okay at ANY age! Nor should you have to deal with bullying AT ANY AGE!

Go into life with humor and kindness...and you may have to look for it. (Alicia, age 58)

Try and leave this world a little better than you found it, and when your turn comes to die, you can die happy in feeling that, at any rate, you have not wasted your time but have done your best. (Lieutenant General Robert Baden-Powell, founder of the worldwide Boy Scout movement and cofounder of the worldwide Girl Guide/ Girl Scout movement)

And as well expressed by one of the local dentists, I may have to get older, but I don't have to grow up or something close to that. (Dr. Tim, age 68)

If you haven't grown up by age 60...you don't have to! (Facebook)

Immaturity never gets old.

Some people call them DECADES—I prefer to call them my "COLLECTED WORKS." (Leigh Standley, 2006)

Laugh like you're 10.
Party like you're 20.
Travel like you're 30.
Think like you're 40.
Advise like you're 50.
Care like you're 60.
Love like you're 70.
(Facebook, Higher Perspective)

Anybody want to touch THAT one?

Collection of random reality and thoughts on aging from my dear friend Mary, age 60-something:

I only can talk / give my opinion on aging. Never had time to reach out to other people. Never really thought about the aging process. But here it goes... You want the time/age I thought... I'm old? Well, around 18-19 years old. Legal! Parents cannot tell me what to do, right? Fun but not fun. Thankful for my parents when I stumbled and got pregnant at 19. You grow/age... You gave life. You age by which path you want to follow (good or bad). Never really question why this person had a little bit of wrinkles. Then another person didn't have that many. Until I got them!

It was by how you cared for your body. Sometimes it was weight gain or weight loss, acne, body aches. List can go on with me the subject of aging. Now at 60-plus, I think back about my mom, how she did it all, the "process of life," and how we age differently. Just "thank" the "Dear Lord" every day you have the gift of life to breathe until he call us home. Aging is "beautiful." Whoever would have thought that I would say those words. The end.

Reminders of important things in the lives of each generation

1928-1945—**Silent Generation / The Greatest Generation**—The Great Depression, WWII, the migration to the West Coast, automobile culture, cigarettes, big band music, swing dance, newsreels at the theaters, and radio.

My dad bought a bright, shiny yellow sports car when he was near 80. And he took us for a ride in his newest midlife crisis acquisition, in the middle of which and going about 70, he laughingly said, "Not bad! I can't feel the gas pedal (from neuropathy)." He sold his new bright-yellow toy shortly after the screaming and yelling stopped.

1946-1964—**Baby Boomers**—Rock 'n' roll, the "American Dream," a TV in every house, mass-produced packaged food, Beatles, Vietnam, Kent State, flower children, civil rights movement, Woodstock, mind-enhancing drugs, corporate America, polio vaccine, Barbie and Ken, vinyls, and equal rights protests.

People born in the '50s have lived in 7 decades, 2 centuries, and 2 millenia. We had the best music, fastest cars, drive-in theaters, soda fountains, and happy days. And we are not even that old yet. We're just that cool. (David Coull, the Fabulous Fifties Group, Facebook, May 6, 2021)

I survived the '60s—TWICE! Well, almost.

Checking out at the store, the young cashier suggested to the much older lady that she should bring her own grocery bags because plastic bags are not good for the environment.

The woman apologized to the young girl and explained, "We didn't have this *green thing* back in my earlier days."

The young clerk responded, "That's our problem today. Your generation did not care enough to save our environment for future generations."

The older lady said that she was right; our generation didn't have the *green thing* in its day. The older lady went on to explain: "Back then, we returned milk bottles, soda bottles, and beer bottles to the store. The store sent them back to the plant to be washed and sterilized and refilled so it could use the same bottles over and over. So they really were recycled.

But we didn't have the *green thing* back in our day. Grocery stores bagged our groceries in brown paper bags that we reused for numerous things. Most memorable besides household garbage bags was the use of brown paper bags as book covers for our schoolbooks. This was to ensure that public property [the book provided for our use by the school] was not defaced by our scribblings. Then we were able to personalize our books on the brown paper bags.

But too bad we didn't do the *green thing* back then. We walked upstairs because we didn't have an escalator in every store and office building. We walked to the grocery store and didn't climb into a 300-horsepower machine every time we had to go two blocks. But she was right. We didn't have the *green thing* in our day.

Back then, we washed the baby's diapers because we didn't have the throwaway kind. We dried clothes on a line, not in an energy-gobbling machine burning up 220 volts. Wind and solar power really did dry our clothes back in our early days.

Kids got hand-me-down clothes from their brothers or sisters, not always brand-new clothing." But that young lady is right. We didn't have the *green thing* back in our day.

Back then, we had one TV or radio in the house—not a TV in every room. And the TV had a small screen the size of a handkerchief [remember them?], not a screen the size of Montana.

In the kitchen, we blended and stirred by hand because we didn't have electric machines to do everything for us.

When we packaged a fragile item to send in the mail, we used wadded-up old newspapers to cushion it, not Styrofoam or plastic bubble wrap.

Back then, we didn't fire up an engine and burn gasoline just to cut the lawn. We used a push mower that ran on human power.

We exercised by working, so we didn't need to go to a health club to run on treadmills that operate on electricity. But she's right; we didn't have the *green thing* back then.

Back then, people took the streetcar or a bus, and kids rode their bikes to school or walked instead of turning their moms into a 24-hour taxi service in the family's $45,000 SUV or van, which costs what a whole house did before the *green thing*.

We had one electrical outlet in a room, not an entire bank of sockets to power a dozen appliances. And we didn't need a computerized gadget to receive a signal beamed from satellites 23,000 miles out in space in order to find the nearest burger joint.

But isn't it sad the current generation laments how wasteful we old folks were just because we didn't have the *green thing* back then?

[Because it's from Facebook,] please forward this on to another selfish old person who needs a lesson in conservation from a smart-ass young person. We don't like being old in the first place, so it doesn't take much to piss us off...especially from a tattooed, multiple-pierced smart-ass who can't make change without the cash register telling them how much. (Terra Barton III, the Fabulous Fifties Group, Facebook, September 11, 2019)

1965–1980—**Gen Xers**—The lost generation, "latchkey kids," "daycare generation," work-life balance, AIDS, and the virtuous midlife crisis.

Forget the sports car and new trophy spouse, for Generation Xers, those 40-55, it's yoga, meditation retreats and keto diets. Many people in their 40s and 50s now simply can't afford an old-school midlife crisis. (Susan Swearingen, *the Wall Street Journal*)

1981-1996—**Millenials**—The "Me, Me, Me Generation" (*Time* magazine), Cabbage Patch dolls, economic prosperity, hip-hop and rap, Columbine, 9/11 and the war on terror, cell phones, the internet, social media, legalization of gay marriage, the Great Recession, young tech gurus, online dating, married to technology and depressed, working smarter and not harder, more idealistic, more confrontational, and into experiences and travel.

Aaron, age 49, commented that "aging sucks," which reflects a generational difference (he's a Gen Xer) but sounds an awful lot like Amanda's.

> Adulting sucks. I do think it's funny and telling that my generation (millennials) made "adulting" a verb. But it's never used in a positive form. It's always "Adulting sucks" or "Adulting is hard." Why are we so pessimistic? Otherwise, I honestly don't think much about aging. I think of time passing but never about getting older very much, if that makes sense. (Amanda, age 39)

Vignette

Amanda is one of my daughters from another mother. She and Ian didn't know they weren't related for real for a very long time in their little lives. She was rather spoiled—she'll admit it—and a very picky eater, and puberty with her and other "daughters" about finished off all of us! However, she has evolved into one of the most admirable wives and mothers that I know. I wanted her to take on the topic of aging because she has MS and I wondered if that might affect her view on it. However, she has one of the most determinably positive attitudes on the unpredictable future and is more than willing to spread around her positivity. I love her.

> I'm looking forward to understanding what retirement means. I'm also looking forward (and scared) to see what our wisdom and teachings bring forth in the younger generation. With social media, I'm not sure people really care about people. They seem to care about animals a lot. But we need to care about people too. (Dr. Matthew, principal, age 40)

Another reason getting older sucks: you get really emotional watching movies you've seen a million times since you were seven, during scenes you never used to get emotional during. Hello, *Dirty Dancing*. (Mia, teacher, age 39)

And yes, 3 of 4 can't be wrong. They must've also made usage of the word *sucks* commonplace!

Just a friendly reminder that the number of millennials that are eligible to vote now exceeds the number of living baby boomers. This country is yours for the taking. (Facebook)

1997–2012—**Gen Z**—"First generation of true digital natives"/self-learners online, seeking truth, freedom of liberal expression, greater openness to understanding differ-ent types of people, mobilization around causes (i.e., Black Lives Matter), truth seekers, rejection of stereotypes, "radically inclusive," into online communities.

2013-present—**Gen Alpha**—COVID-19
(**Pew Research Center**; Kristen Fuller, MD, "From Baby Boomers to Gen Z," *Psychology Today*; Ian, age 39; Tracy Francis and Fernanda Hoefel, **McKinsey & Company**, Nov. 12, 2018; "Generational Difference Chart," **wmfc.org**)
(Please note that there are some disagreements on the exact years of these and that this reflects things which have occurred during their "time.")

Being an adult is the **dumbest** thing I have EVER done.

"When you think of becoming older or parents becoming older, what comes to mind?" I asked Ian.
"Nothing good. I worry about declining health, limited mobility, loss of independence, and the inevitable need for continuous care."
"What about the Golden Years?"

"It's a pipe dream. Gramom and Grampy used to have a pillow that said 'Screw the Golden Years,'" said Ian, age 39.

This is from MY Ian, my Sunshine Boy. Life has tainted his perspective. He is from the "sucks" generation unfortunately. I still have hope that things will brighten for them.

Some people are old at 18, and some are young at 90. Time is a concept that humans created. (Facebook)

Old age is 50 years older than I am. (Oliver Wendell Holmes Jr., former associate justice of the Supreme Court of the United States)

I think the proper term for "senior" women should be Queen-agers. That is all. Carry on. (Facebook)

Don't blink
Just like that you're six years old and you take a nap and you
Wake up and you're twenty-five and your high school sweetheart becomes your wife
Don't blink
You just might miss your babies growing like mine did
Turning into moms and dads next thing you know your "better half"
Of fifty years is there in bed
And you're praying God takes you instead
Trust me friend a hundred years goes faster than you think
So don't blink.
(**Kenny Chesney**, American singer/songwriter, "Don't Blink")

I try to take one day at a time...but lately several days have attacked me at once! (Facebook)

Morning is God's way of saying, "One more time, go make a difference, touch a heart, encourage a mind, inspire a soul, and enjoy the day." (Facebook; writer's note—Whatever age you are!)

Life is short. Break the rules. Forgive quickly. Kiss slowly. Love truly. Laugh uncontrollably, and never regret ANYTHING that makes you smile. (Mark Twain, American writer)

We all share the same lifetime. Let's be nice to each other. (Facebook)

Age is irrelevant. Ask me how many sunsets I've seen, hearts I've loved, trips I've taken, or concerts I've been to. THAT'S how old I am. (Facebook)

Life really does begin at forty. Up until then, you are just doing research. (Facebook)

I didn't reach my athletic peak until I was 43.
I didn't write my first book until I was 44.
I didn't start my podcast until I was 45.
At 30, I thought my life was over.
At 52, I know it's just beginning.
(Facebook)

Life is short. If you can't laugh at yourself, call me. I will. (Facebook)

Here's to all my girlfriends who will help me cause trouble in the nursing home. (Facebook)

Someday we old folks will use cursive writing as a secret code! (Facebook)

Never be a prisoner of your past. It was just a lesson, not a life sentence. (Facebook)

I'm thankful I only have to grow old once. I don't think I could do it twice. (Facebook)

Old age isn't easy, but I'm not ready for the alternative! (Sallie, 73)

You're here, so accept it. Make it look good and move on. (Diana, age 73)

Here's my view on aging. Don't do it, but if you have to, do it with acceptance and a smile. Set a good example for the kids. (Kathy, age 84; writer's note—Kathy, you know what the alternative is if you don't do it...)

Vignette

I nominated Kathy for sainthood probably 10 years into our almost-40-year relationship. She was Ian's babysitter extraordinaire. She walked him downtown so frequently to the library, the county extension office, and the stores that, at age 2 or 3, he knew more people than I did. And they knew him! During the many years, our families merged with some on the West Coast and others on the East. And Kathy remained "our Kathy"—steadfast, sincere, positive, supportive, happy, and somewhere between aunt / mother / best friend. In my mind, she doesn't age—she can't. We won't let her.

There exists on YouTube a WONDERFUL (rated R for language; take it in context) video done by our community's TV claim to fame (*A Million Little Things*). And not because he's our native son, but because it's just plain good! Please check out the whole thing if you have a chance. It's Sam Pancake's (real given name—honestly!) plea to "**respect gay elders**," a cry from the heart. He speaks of the toll of HIV and AIDS on gay men his age before launching into an impassioned plea about ageism in the gay community. Sam watched a lot of his friends die in the 1990s as they paved the way for gays who followed them to have a much more comfortable life. However, when this young 30 something upstart made one too many snide remarks to Sam, like "I'd rather be dead than old," instead of granting his wish, Sam sprang on him, like a stretched rubber band, in a "Respect your elders who made life easy for you, babycakes" type lecture. And it's been a hit! (Tracy Gilchrist, January 29, 2020)

Wonder if the kid gets it yet? In fact, I wonder if he realizes that Greg Louganis, 1984 and 1988 Olympic gold medalist (Johnny Dodd, *People* magazine, January 27, 2020);

Neil Patrick Harris, actor; Ellen DeGeneres, American comedian; and Elton John, singer extraordinaire, along with many other brave "old" people, did a lot to allow him the comforts of being an aging gay man in 2020?

Do we have to know who's gay and who's straight? Can't we just love everybody and judge them by the car they drive? (Ellen DeGeneres, 60-something, comedian, talk show host, dancer, humanitarian, social rights activist, and animal rights activist)

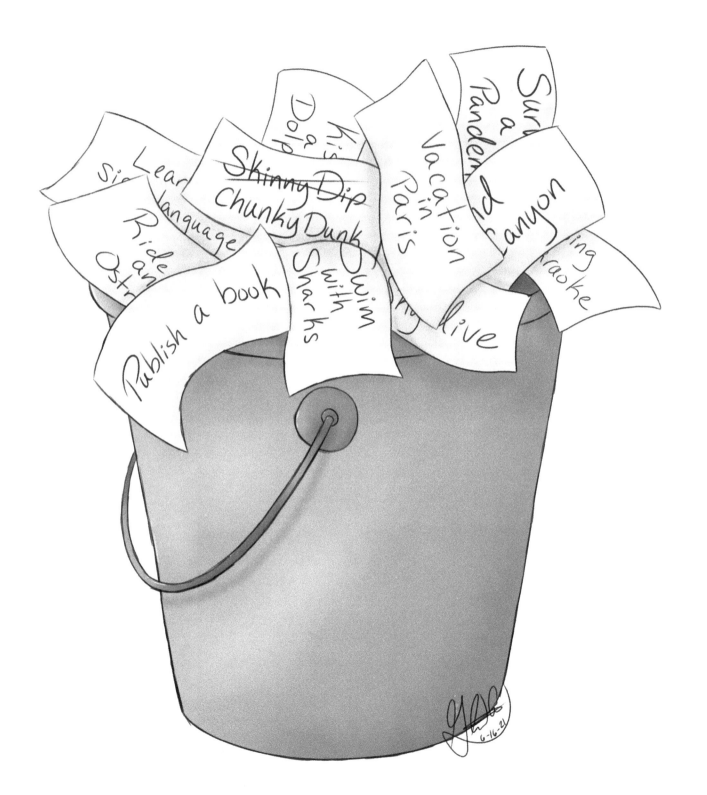

Soul

Tibetan Proverb—The secret to living well and longer is to eat half, walk double, laugh triple, and love without measure. (Facebook)

Dear God, if today I lose my hope, please remind me that Your plans are better than my dreams. (Facebook)

Sometimes our lives have to be completely shaken up, changed, and rearranged to relocate us to the place we're meant to be. (Mandy Hale, author)

Enjoy the little things in life because one day you'll look back and realize they were the big things. (Facebook)

At the end of life, what really matters is not what we had, but what we built; not what we got, but what we shared; not our competence, but our character; and not our success, but our significance. Live a life that matters. Live a life of love. (John Tesh, American pianist, composer, and radio host)

May the road rise up to meet you.
May the wind be always at your back.
May the sun shine warm upon your face.

And rains fall soft upon your fields.
And, until we meet again,
May God hold you in the palm of his hand.
(Irish Blessing)

People come and go in your life. But the right ones will always stay. (Facebook) (writer's note—gently shake off the ones who are wrong.)

Stay close to people who feel like sunlight. (Facebook)

As you get older, you care less about what people think and more about being true to yourself. I like to get my hair done to look and feel beautiful on the outside and to be empathetic toward others to feel good inside. Every day, think of things you are grateful for to keep anxiety away. (Roz, graphic artist, age 55)

I look forward to not caring as much about what people think. (Ian, vice president, public relations, age 39)

Treasure love for your family, love for your spouse, and love for your friends. Appreciate what you have. Don't treat your spouse or significant other INsignificantly!

My doctor asked if any members of my family suffered from insanity. I said, "Nope, we all seem to enjoy it." (RUSAFU—Rude, Sarcastic, Funny Thoughts, Quotes, and Sayings)

Don't judge me by my relatives. If you met my family, you'd understand.

It's okay to cut ties with toxic family members. (Facebook)

Love is rare. Grab it.
Anger is bad. Dump it.
Fear is awful. Face it.

Memories are sweet. Cherish them.
Life is short, Live it!
(Facebook)

Consider this: Instead of a bucket list of things we want to do before we die that can set us up for disappointment, what about having a bucket into which you toss notes on new or exceptional things you've done! My bucket is from the beach and had 32 ounces of rum punch in it...which I drank...all by myself. And that was my first note! OOO, and now I can add writing a book!

Stop apologizing.

You don't have to say sorry for how you laugh, how you dress, how you do your hair, how you do your makeup, how you speak.
You don't have to be sorry for being yourself. Do it fearlessly. It's time to accept this is you, and you gotta spend the rest of your life with you. So start loving your sarcasm, your awkwardness, your weirdness, your peculiar habits, your unique sense of humor, your voice, your talents, your everything. It will make your life so much easier to simply be yourself. (Facebook)

How many of you still have food from your 1999/2000 stockpile for the computer "glitch"? No, wait, I CAN'T be the only one!

How come you never see those great cars like the Boss Mustang, or the T-Bird with the opera windows, or the T-sunroof Corvettes, or the Volkswagen bugs on the streets anymore? Huh? They'd be HOW old? NOOOO! They weren't EVER supposed to age! Maybe that's why I've only seen them on TV for a long time.

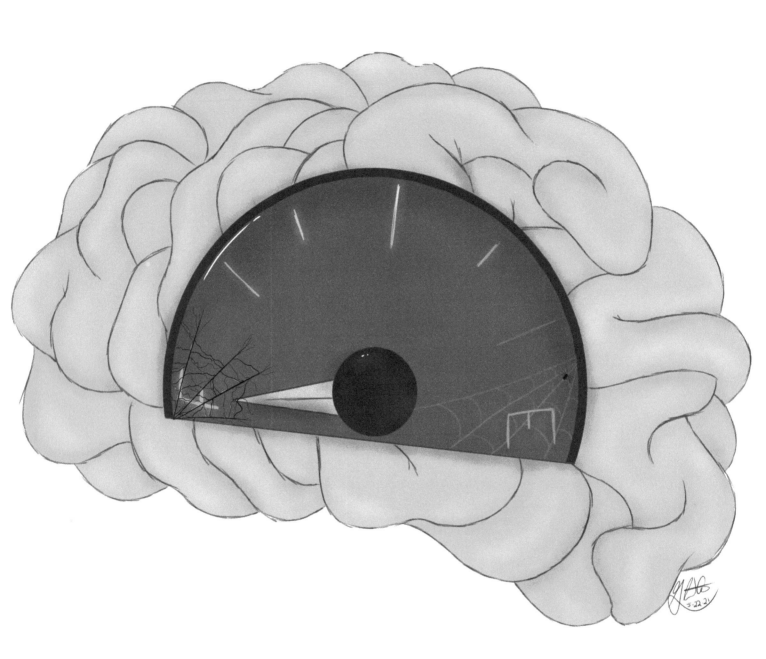

Remaining Wisdom

No one is going to stand up at your funeral and say, "They had a really expensive couch and great shoes." Don't make life about stuff. (Facebook)

What a wonderful life I've had! I only wish I'd realized it sooner. (Colette, French author)

Life humbles you as you age. You realize how much time you wasted on nonsense. (Facebook)

Live your life and forget your age. (Facebook)

All I know about tomorrow is that God will rise before the sun.

I'm too old for games, too tired to pretend, and too wise for lies. (Facebook)

Don't think of us as getting older. Think of us as flower children gone to seed!

"You're still a rock star," I whisper to myself as I take my multivitamin and get in bed at 9. (Facebook)

The fact is that the real rise to the top is a lot easier than it sounds. Just let go of the idea that you need to climb somewhere or something, and concentrate on lifting and inspiring others along their journey. When you stop focusing on yourself, you end up finding extraordinary joy in watching others' dreams take flight. (Suzy Toronto, *Life Is All About How You Handle Plan B*)

These are the end-all recommendations for staving off ill effects of aging, from "Spring Clean Your Brain!" by Paula Spencer Scott in *Parade*, April 11, 2021: She quotes Daniel Levitin, neuroscientist and author of *Successful Aging* that we must, Number 1, "be brave and fight the tendencies to reject trying new things." Number 2 is to "respect our biorhythms—in bed at the same time every night, up at the same time every day. Even going off these times by one hour can throw off our whole systems by one week or more." David Perlmutter, MD, author of *Brain Wash* recommends, Number Three, meditating.

What about "box breathing"? First slowly exhale through your mouth counting to 4. Second breathe in through your nose counting to 4. Third hold breath counting to four. Fourth exhale through mouth counting to 4. Repeat until you feel calmer.

Number 4, oh, he also suggests growing your own. Gardening, especially greens, which may slow cognitive decline, and communing with nature may reduce anxiety. Gary Small, MD, director of the UCLA Longevity Center and coauthor of *The Small Guide to Alzheimer's Disease*, gives the big whammy with, Number 5, "exercise making the brain BIGGER, especially in areas of memory! And bigger is better." He also recommends dietary EXchanges, like switching out ice cream with Greek yogurt. His suggestion of adding curcumin (in turmeric) for memory did not sit well with my digestion, so be conscious of these changes. Number 6, "belly laugh to release endorphins and reduce stress," says Lisa Mosconi, neuroscientist and director of the Weill Cornell Medicine Women's Brain Initiative and author of *The XX Brain*. And Number 7, "practice gratitude because it provides a mood boost," according to Sarah Lenz Lock, executive director of the Global Council on Brain Health.

Marriage, engagement, pregnancy, a new child are all amazing things to celebrate; but they are not the only things. Don't forget to celebrate your friend who ran a marathon, who left a toxic relationship, who went back to school, who is taking steps to heal from trauma! (Facebook)

The thing is, when people fall for somebody, it feels exactly the same as it did when you were 16. It doesn't feel any different physically or mentally. People sometimes need to be reminded of that. (Jean Smart, American actor)

If you remember anything of me after I leave this world, remember that I loved even when it was foolish, that I cared even when it was unwanted. When my body is gone, remember my heart. (Facebook)

The tongue has no bones but is strong enough to break a heart. So be careful with your words. (Amanda Rudisill, Facebook)

So what will my personal beauty philosophy be as I get older? To strive for an A in physical perfection would require me to think about myself too much, which is boring to me and certainly to others. I'd become a woman consumed by my shortfalls, by my physical imperfections-a glass half empty, not half full. Instead, I want to wear my age with grace, confidence, and contentedness. I expect there will be many Cs but also, I hope a couple of As and Bs for character, humor, and personality... Our physical attributes cannot outrun the passage of time. But no woman at any age can look unattractive or old if she is laughing, smiling, or engaged with others. (Diane Pascoe, American author, *Life Isn't Perfect, But My Lipstick Is*)

This is from Ellen van der Molen (as posted to Facebook by Starlette Tolver, consultant)

I asked a friend who has crossed 70 and is heading toward 80 what sort of changes she is feeling in herself.

She sent me the following:

1. After loving my parents, my siblings, my spouse, my children, and my friends, I have now started loving myself.
2. I have realized that I am not "Atlas." The world does not rest on my shoulders.
3. I have stopped bargaining with vegetable and fruit vendors. A few pennies more is not going to break me, but it might help the poor fellow save for his daughter's school fees.
4. I leave my waitress a big tip. The extra money might bring a smile to her face. She is toiling much harder for a living than I am.
5. I stopped telling the elderly that they've already narrated that story many times. The story makes them walk down memory lane and relive their past.
6. I have learned not to correct people even when I know they are wrong. The onus of making everyone perfect is not on me. Peace is more precious than perfection.
7. I give compliments freely and generously. Compliments are a mood enhancer not only for the recipient but also for me. And a small tip for the recipient of a compliment—never, NEVER turn it down. Just say, "Thank you."
8. I have learned not to bother about a crease or a spot on my shirt. Personality speaks louder than appearances.
9. I walk away from people who don't value me. They may not know my worth, but I do.
10. I remain cool when someone plays dirty to outrun me in the rat race. I am not a rat, and neither am I in any race.
11. I am learning not to be embarrassed by my emotions. It's my emotions that make me human.
12. I have learned that it's better to drop the ego than to break a relationship. My ego will keep me aloof whereas, with relation-ships, I will never be alone.

13. I have learned to live each day as if it's the last. After all, it might be the last.
14. I am doing what makes me happy. I am responsible for my happiness, and I owe it to myself. Happiness is a choice. You can be happy at any time. Just choose to be!

Excerpted from some of Steve Jobs' last words:

Your true inner happiness does not come from the material things of this world. Whether you're flying first class, or economy class—if the plane crashes, you crash with it. The results will be the same.

If the house we live in is 300 square meters, or 3000 square meters—the loneliness is the same. So, I hope you understand that, when you have friends or someone to talk to, this is true happiness!

The six best doctors in the world:

1. Sunlight
2. Rest
3. Exercise
4. Diet
5. Self-Confidence
6. Friends

Keep them in all stages of life and enjoy a healthy life.

Whichever stage in life we are at right now, with time, we will face the day when the curtain comes down.

Treat yourself well. Cherish others. (Steve Jobs, American business magnate)

Perhaps one has to be very old before one learns how to be amused rather than shocked. (Pearl S. Buck, West Virginia, American author; writer's note—You know, Ms. Pearl, I believe you're onto something there. It's much easier to snicker under a mask in a situation where the teacher in me would previously possibly have felt the need to intervene. I just hope my eyes don't give me away. Plus, I just don't give a flying fig as much anymore.)

Ten Things to Remember for a Wonderful Wacky Life

#10 Think big. If that doesn't work, think bigger.
#9 If you want rainbows, you gotta have rain.
#8 When life become a roller coaster, climb into the front seat, throw your arms in the air, and enjoy the ride.
#7 Inches, ages, and sizes don't tell you anything about the amazing woman (people) inside.
#6 When life gives you a second chance, take it.
#5 Pretending to be a normal person day after day is exhausting.
#4 Age is nothing but a state of mind.
#3 Art does not have to match your sofa.
#2 Always color outside the lines.
And the #1 thing to always remember and never, ever forget is this: **Life is all about how you handle Plan B.**
(Suzy Toronto, *Life Is All About How You Handle Plan B*)

We've learned how to make a living but not a life. And always remember, life is not measured by the number of breaths we take but by those moments that take our breath away. (George Carlin, 1937-2008, Facebook)

Don't forget those SENIOR DISCOUNTS! Some stores offer a certain percentage off on a particular day of the week. Mark your calendars if you're flexible enough to shop whenever you want. Others offer a standing percent off for seniors all the time or a senior menu, i.e., IHOP. These may be smaller portions so be aware, although that may be what you prefer anyway. Or you can get the larger portion and a carryout box when your meal is served and just divide the meal in half to enjoy half at the restaurant and half at home!

SUBSCRIBE TO **AARP**! They have all kinds of good stuff, discounts, tips, and articles all relevant to the "older crowd." Here are some of my recent finds:

Five Popular Grocery Items That Will Cost You More This Summer

1. Chicken wings—Chicken thighs will be cheaper this year.
2. Bacon—Rising feed and labor costs are showing up.
3. Fresh fruits (boo)—You'll be facing increasing labor and transportation costs. Good reasons to shop locally and support farm gardens in your neighborhood.
4. Beef—We are at the will of rising processing and packaging costs...AND hacking of packaging companies! Think veggie products. We recently tried the new veggie burgers, and they were super!
5. Milk—Whole milk is up 7.2 percent over last year; lower fat milk is up 3.2 percent. But ice cream is DOWN 2.6, and cheese is down 1.4. (Writer's note: HOORAY! It's gonna be a grilled cheese and ice cream kind of summer!)

(John Waggoner, **AARP**, June 10, 2021)

The Daily Five Essentials to Keep in Your Medicine Cabinet After 50

1. Pain relievers—Acetaminophen (Tylenol) is safest.
2. Heartburn helpers—Chewable calcium carbonate, you know, the ones that have been around for YEARS (Tums)!
3. Allergy alleviators—Cetirizine (Zyrtec) or loratadine (Claritin). (Writer's note: I inserted brand names because...it's confusing. I have found that most of the generics work as well as the brand name products. Just read the labels to be sure they will not adversely react with any of your other medicines or conditions. Also, they may make you sleepy. Nighttime is probably a better time to take them.)
4. Cold and cough—Hot tea with honey, ice water, OR a single ingredient over-the-counter medication(to reduce the side effects).
5. First aid fixes—Adhesive bandages, gauze, antibiotic ointment, calamine lotion, hydrocortisone cream. (Writer's note: Watch that tapes don't tear tender skin! Skin thins as we age. Companies make skin-sensitive bandages. Also, keep a little package

of sanitary pads in the event of a bloody incident, like a fall where one's head hits concrete; I wish I'd known this tip then. Details will be included in Book 2.)

(Rachel Nania, **AARP**, June 3, 2021)

The Daily Seven Superfoods to Eat After 50

1. Berries
2. Dark-green leafy vegetables
3. Seafood
4. Nuts and seeds
5. Cottage cheese
6. Bean and legumes

(Alison Gwinn, **AARP**, June 3, 2021)

Seven Common Health Problems That Can Strike After 50

1. High blood pressure
2. High cholesterol
3. Diabetes
4. Arthritis
5. Osteoporosis
6. Cancer
7. Anxiety/depression

(Rachel Nania, **AARP**, May 18, 2021)

Warning

When I am an old woman I shall wear purple
With a red hat which doesn't go, and doesn't suit me
And I shall spend my pension on brandy and summer gloves
And satin sandals, and say we've no money for butter.
I shall sit down on the pavement when I'm tired
And gobble up samples in shops and press alarm bells
And run my stick along the public railings
And make up for the sobriety of my youth.
I shall go out in my slippers in the rain
And pick flowers in other people's gardens
And learn to spit.

You can wear terrible shirts and grow more fat
And eat three pounds of sausages at a go
Or only bread and pickle for a week
And hoard pens and pencils and beermats and things in boxes.

But now we must have clothes that keep us dry
And pay our rent and not swear in the street
And set a good example for the children.
We must have friends to dinner and read the papers

But maybe I ought to practice a little now?
So people who know me are not too shocked and surprised
When suddenly I am old, and start to wear purple.

(From the Scottish Poetry Library by Jenny Joseph)

And having survived COVID-19, the pandemic of 2020/21/22, if you're reading this, take away this one thing—hand sanitizer takes off permanent marker.

Index and Health References

About the Author

Robin is retired from the West Virginia Schools for the Deaf and the Blind, where she served students in all areas of the curriculum. She holds undergraduate and graduate degrees in education. She has been active with youth in the community and church and has participated in programs and organizations focusing on the rights of disabled adults and children. She enjoys treasure hunting through yard sales, bargain stores, and online retailers. Robin lives in Romney, West Virginia, with her husband, Kenny, and three cat kids, although she feels her soul comes to rest at the beach. She has traveled extensively in the US and in Europe, where she most recently toured a hospital in Germany after one-too-many *interesting* experiences. (See book number 2—*Trips, Travels, Travails with the Ayers*—or something like that.)

CPSIA information can be obtained
at www.ICGtesting.com
Printed in the USA
BVHW022247070522
636437BV00017B/765